PRACTICAL N

Practical Neonatal Paediatrics

R.J.K.BROWN
M.B. F.R.C.P. D.C.H.
Consultant Paediatrician to the Middlesex Hospital,
Queen Elizabeth Hospital for Children, London
and the Hackney Hospital

H.B.VALMAN
M.D. F.R.C.P. D.C.H. D.R.C.O.G.
Consultant Paediatrician to
Northwick Park Hospital and Clinical Research Centre,
Harrow, Middlesex

FOREWORD BY
SIR STANLEY G. CLAYTON
M.D. M.S.(Lond.) F.R.C.S. F.R.C.O.G.
Past President of the Royal College of
Obstetricians and Gynaecologists.
Professor Emeritus of Obstetrics and Gynaecology,
King's College Hospital Medical School,
University of London.
Honorary Consulting Surgeon,
Queen Charlotte's Hospital

FOURTH EDITION

BLACKWELL SCIENTIFIC PUBLICATIONS
OXFORD LONDON EDINBURGH MELBOURNE

Osney Mead, Oxford OX2 0EL
8 John Street, London WC1N 2ES
9 Forrest Road, Edinburgh EH1 2QM
214 Berkeley Street, Carlton
Victoria 3053, Australia

First published 1971
Italian edition 1971
Second edition 1973
Third edition 1975
Fourth edition 1979

British Library Cataloguing in Publication Data

Brown, Roderick John Kilner
Practical neonatal paediatrics. – 4th ed.
1. Infants (Newborn) – Diseases
I. Title II. Valman, Hyman Bernard
618.9′201 RJ254

ISBN 0–632–00556–4

Distributed in U.S.A. by
Blackwell Mosby Book Distributors
11830 Westline Industrial Drive
St Louis, Missouri 63141,
in Canada by
Blackwell Mosby Book Distributors
86 Northline Road, Toronto
Ontario, M4B 3E5,
and in Australia by
Blackwell Scientific Book Distributors
214 Berkeley Street, Carlton
Victoria 3053

Set in VIP Times by Bishopsgate Press Ltd., London
Printed and bound in Great Britain by
Billing & Sons Ltd.
Guildford, London and Worcester

Contents

Contents

Foreword

As an obstetrician I welcome the publication of this book because it exactly fulfils the purpose stated in the preface—to give practical advice and instruction to those who are responsible for the day to day care of the newborn infant. It sets out the management of each problem clearly and, although it never departs far from practical considerations, basic explanations are never lacking. It is a tribute to the concise good style of the text that it is so easily readable when so much has been included.

As an introduction to the subject for those starting paediatrics it should be invaluable, and I judge it to be particularly suitable for obstetricians, both junior and senior, who often need immediate guidance and yet lack paediatric experience.

Whether the obstetric staff or the staff of the children's department should be primarily responsible for the management of the newborn child is a matter of no importance, provided that they cooperate to give good care, and this book will greatly help them to achieve that.

STANLEY G. CLAYTON

Preface to the fourth edition

In revising for the fourth edition we have deliberately set out to preserve the character of this book as an easily readable guide rather than a textbook. Inevitably much detail has to be omitted in the interests of brevity.

Considerable changes have been made in most of the chapters to include the large number of recent advances in the care of the newborn.

We are grateful to Dr. H.V.L. Finlay for his meticulous reading of the draft of the present and previous editions and many helpful suggestions. We thank Dr. Mary Cummins for writing the section on intravenous feeding.

Preface to the third edition

The object of this book is to provide the paediatric house physician, obstetric house surgeon, midwife and medical student with easily accessible information on the management of the newborn infant. No previous paediatric experience is assumed and the chapters are arranged according to gross presenting features. The methods described are those practised at the Middlesex, Northwick Park and Hackney Hospitals and the Queen Elizabeth Hospital for Children, London. We have used the word 'practical' in the title in the sense that the methods can be practised with the resources available at most district hospitals. Apart from the few babies who require transfer to specialised units, we consider that these methods provide optimum care. With few exceptions, details of technical procedures have not been included as we believe these should be taught and supervised personally. Each chapter has been written to help with a particular clinical problem and some repetition has been unavoidable. Most of the material has been previously published in the standard textbooks and journals and we have attempted to present a simplified even if dogmatic, approach.

Acknowledgements

In order to make this book a practical guide we have simplified the text by omitting references. Most of the material has been derived from our teachers, our nursing and medical colleagues and the standard textbooks and journals. We thank all those who have contributed; it is impossible to mention each one individually.

We are extremely grateful to Professor Sir Stanley G. Clayton for writing the foreword.

We are grateful to Miss D.J. Davis, Dr R. Blowers and Dr H.V.L. Finlay for constructive criticism and Dr F.E. Hytten for help with the orientation of Chapter 1. We thank Dr C.O. Carter for advising on the preparation of the table on congenital abnormalities. We are grateful to the authors and publishers who have allowed us to reproduce material. We thank Mr Per Saugman for encouraging us to prepare this fourth edition so shortly after the third and enabling us to include many recent advances.

Acknowledgements

CHAPTER ONE

The 'At Risk' Infant

OBJECT

To identify the infant at special risk of death or disease before, during or after delivery.

Adverse factors

At the first visit adverse factors should be sought including previous obstetric problems, elderly primigravidy, grand multigravidy, hypertension, a height below 1.5 m and hereditary disease in the family.

Delay in attending for the first antenatal visit and failure to keep appointments for the antenatal clinic are associated with an increased perinatal mortality.

The perinatal mortality is the number of stillbirths and 1st week deaths in 1000 total births. The combined figures for 1975 and 1976 in England and Wales was 14.5 in social classes I and II and 21.7 in social classes IV and V. Illegitimacy is associated with a high perinatal mortality. These adverse social factors can be determined early in pregnancy.

FETOPLACENTAL INSUFFICIENCY

The fetus may grow poorly and become anoxic which may cause death before or during labour. The fetus and placenta should be considered as one unit as tests of function usually do not separate the effect of each part. Impaired fetoplacental function should be considered if there is hypertension, vaginal bleeding, or postmaturity. Vaginal bleeding at any stage of pregnancy always indicates that there is a potential hazard to the fetus. There is a higher incidence of poor fetal growth in first pregnancies and occasionally there is a history of recurrent abortion or a previous infant with intrauterine malnutrition. Cigarette smoking causes poor fetal growth and increased perinatal mortality. If the mother gains less than 0.5 kg/week over a 3-week period during the final 3 months of pregnancy, and is not vomiting or dieting, inadequate fetal growth should be considered.

A reliable estimate of the gestational age of the fetus is needed before retarded growth can be diagnosed. Maturity of the fetus is particularly difficult to assess if the mother is unsure of the dates of her last menstrual period, if the cycle is irregular or if she has recently stopped taking an oral contraceptive. Maturity can be accurately assessed by two clinical examinations by the same observer within the first 16 weeks of pregnancy.

The gestational age, size of the fetus and rate of growth can be confirmed by serial measurements of the biparietal diameter of the fetal skull by ultrasound but this method is only accurate in the first 32 weeks. Recently, accuracy has been increased by measuring the biparietal to thoracic diameter and by measuring liver size as this is an early indicator of fetal malnutrition. Interference with brain growth is relatively late compared with other organs. Ultrasound can give misleading results if the technical skill of the operator is faulty.

The appearance of fetal ossification centres is not an accurate method of assessing maturing as there is considerable normal variation.

Estimation of the lecithin: sphingomyelin (L/S) ratio in the amniotic fluid can predict the functional maturity of the fetal lung. If the ratio is more than 2:1 the infant is unlikely to develop respiratory distress syndrome (see p.65) but there is a high risk if the ratio is less than 1.5:1. The rise in the ratio is accelerated in maternal hypertension and may be misleading in diabetes mellitus, but is the single and most useful investigation (see p.106). The L/S ratio may be elevated when the fetus has been subjected to stress by hypertension, antepartum haemorrhage or prolonged rupture of the membranes and may also be raised by giving betamethasone to the mother for at least 24 h before delivery. There is an increase in the perinatal mortality if a mother with hypertension receives betamethasone.

None of the tests to confirm fetoplacental function are completely reliable but falling levels of maternal urinary oestriol or changes in the levels of certain enzymes in the mother's serum, for example fetal placental lactogen, may be the only indicators that fetal death is imminent and that there is need for urgent delivery. These tests cannot be interpreted without an accurate gestational age assessment.

During labour a fetus with or without previous evidence of fetoplacental insufficiency may show signs suggestive of anoxia such as alterations in the heart rate or meconium staining of the liquor. This may be due to placental insufficiency but the possibility of compression of the umbilical cord or the effect of drugs given to the mother should be considered. Characteristic patterns of fetal heart rate during and between uterine contractions, recorded using a monitor with applicators on the mother's abdomen, can help to determine the cause and severity of the anoxia.

If there is doubt about the significance of the fetal heart rate recording confirmatory evidence can be provided by taking a sample of blood from the scalp of the fetus and measuring the pH. This shows the severity of the anoxia and whether immediate delivery is indicated.

An infant born after intrauterine malnutrition weighs less than would be expected from the gestational age. These babies are below the 10th centile for gestational age and are called light-for-dates infants (see pp.43,108).They are particularly susceptible to hypoglycaemia in the first 72 h of life and this can result in permanent brain damage if it is symptomatic and prolonged (see p.63). The placenta usually appears macroscopically *normal* and its weight is in proportion to the size of the infant. (The placental weight is normally about one-sixth of the weight of the baby.)

PRE-TERM INFANTS

Infants born before the end of the 37th week of gestation are called pre-term infants. If the mother is uncertain of the dates of her last menstrual period there is a danger that labour will be induced too early and the infant will be subject to the dangers of prematurity. Premature onset of labour is common in twin pregnancies and there are additional hazards of relatively low birth weights compared with singletons and frequently an abnormal presentation. Infants with congenital abnormalities are often born prematurely. Induction of labour before term may be necessary due to an antepartum haemorrhage, hypertension or placental insufficiency. In diabetes mellitus or rhesus incompatibility labour may be induced early to prevent a stillbirth.

FETAL ANOMALY

This is more common if the mother is less than 16 years or over 35 years of age. There may be a family history or the parents may live in an area with a relatively high incidence of a particular anomaly, for example, myelomeningocoele in South Wales. If the uterine size appears to be too large for the length of gestation there may be twins or polyhydramnios, which in some cases is associated with fetal abnormalities, especially defects in the central nervous system and high alimentary tract obstruction. A radiograph or ultrasound examination will exclude twins and may demonstrate a fetal anomaly. Alternatively the uterus may be too small for the gestational age due to an abnormal fetus with retarded growth rate. It may be helpful to estimate the serum rubella and cytomegalovirus antibody titres and to perform a serum toxoplasma dye test. Amniocentesis with a chromosome study of the cultured cells may be of value in selected patients, for example, mothers who have previously had infants with trisomy 21 or those over 40 years.

Raised levels of alphafetoprotein are found in the amniotic fluid when the fetus has anencephaly or an open myelomeningocoele (see p.33). In some hospitals *plasma* alphafetoprotein levels are measured in all mothers at the 12th week of gestation. The level in amniotic fluid is estimated and an ultrasound examination is performed in those mothers with a raised plasma level who wish to have these investigations.

Specific causes

INFECTIONS

Immunoglobulins are specialised proteins carrying antibody function. Maternal IgM does not cross the placenta and a high serum IgM level in the infant at birth is a valuable indication of an intrauterine infection. In contrast IgG crosses the placenta and the infant's serum level at birth is proportional to the maternal serum level. A raised serum antibody titre in a newborn infant may be due to maternal antibody which has passed across the placenta. If the raised specific serum antibody, for example to rubella, in the infant consists of IgM, the fetus has had an active infection with that virus *in utero*.

Rubella virus transmitted during the first 4 months of pregnancy may injure the fetus and interfere with the development of various organs, the type and severity of the injury depending upon the gestational age when the mother was infected. The risk has varied between 10 and 25% in most recorded epidemics (see p.38). Recent evidence suggests that congenital rubella starting after the first 4 months of pregnancy can affect organs already developed causing, for example, nerve deafness. If a woman has a rash in early pregnancy whether it is typical or atypical of rubella or she has had contact with rubella, a clotted venous blood sample should be taken as a matter of urgency and the problem discussed with the microbiologist. It may be necessary to consider therapeutic abortion. The value of gamma globulin is unproven and we do not recommend it. Infants with congenital rubella may excrete the virus in the nasopharyngeal secretions and urine, and are potentially infectious to nursing or medical staff who may be in the early stages of pregnancy.

In some areas girls are being immunised routinely with live, attenuated rubella vaccine at the age of 13 years. If vaccine is given later, conception should be avoided for at least 2 months. If routine determination of serum rubella antibody titre is available at the first antenatal visit, it shows whether the mother is susceptible to infection with rubella.

This is helpful in management if the mother has a rash subsequently or is in contact with a patient with rubella.

Cytomegalovirus (CMV) and toxoplasmosis may produce somewhat similar effects on the fetus. The presence of active cytomegalovirus infection in the mother will probably be unsuspected, but the diagnosis of toxoplasmosis may be considered in the mother if she has an illness simulating infectious mononucleosis, especially when the family has a domestic cat. The diagnosis can be confirmed by a rising titre of the serum toxoplasma dye test.

DRUGS

The fetal abnormalities caused by thalidomide are a reminder that drugs should be avoided in pregnancy if possible and new drugs should not be given.

X-RAYS

No diagnostic radiographs should be taken during pregnancy without pressing clinical reasons as there is a risk of teratogenic effects, particularly in early pregnancy.

BIRTH TRAUMA

The most common reason is that the infant's head is disproportionately large for the pelvic outlet. The mother who has had very large infants previously or whose height is less than 1.5 m is at special risk of a difficult delivery with the possibility of birth trauma to the infant. An abnormal presentation, long labour or precipitate delivery predispose to cerebral birth trauma. Breech delivery may be hazardous especially in the primiparous mother. Precipitate delivery is particularly dangerous to a low birth weight infant.

RHESUS INCOMPATIBILITY

Affected infants may be stillborn, grossly oedematous (hydrops fetalis), severely or moderately jaundiced soon after birth, or liable to become anaemic during the first few weeks after birth (see p.93).

Cells from the fetus may pass into the mother's circulation when the placenta begins to tear away from its attachment to the uterine wall, especially during labour. If the mother is rhesus negative and the fetus rhesus positive, the rhesus positive fetal red cells may stimulate the production of antibodies by the mother. These antibodies can be detected in the maternal serum and during a subsequent pregnancy will pass back across the placenta into the fetus causing haemolysis of the red cells and anaemia if the fetus is rhesus positive. Since transfer of the fetal cells across the placenta occurs especially during labour, these cells can be destroyed, preventing the disease in subsequent infants, by giving all rhesus negative mothers with rhesus positive infants an injection of anti-D antibody shortly after delivery. This preventative measure is not effective if antibodies were already present during the pregnancy.

All rhesus negative mothers should have antibody titres estimated at 12, 28, 32 and 36 weeks of pregnancy. A rising titre suggests that the fetus is affected but neither a rise nor a lack of rise in titre is always a reliable guide to the state of the fetus. If a previous infant has been affected, the father's genotype may help to predict the chances of a further fetus being affected. If the father is heterozygous there is a one in two chance of each subsequent fetus being rhesus positive. Raised pigment levels in the liquor obtained by amniocentesis at about 32 and 34 weeks of pregnancy may predict the presence of a severely affected infant and the need for early delivery. This investigation may also save an unaffected infant from being delivered early with unnecessary dangers of prematurity. Estimation of the L/S ratio on part of the same specimen may help to determine the risk of induction of labour against the risk of conservative management.

If a previous sibling has been severely affected or stillborn due to rhesus incompatibility, the possibility of intrauterine transfusion of the fetus should be considered by referring the mother to the regional rhesus centre. Mothers with an antibody titre of more than 1 in 16 at any stage of pregnancy should also be referred to the centre.

If a previous infant has been severely affected and there is evidence that the present fetus is also affected, suitable blood for exchange transfusion should be available at the time of delivery (see p.89). The criteria for exchange transfusions are still controversial and will vary in different centres. The following recommendations are based on our own experience. Immediate exchange transfusions to raise the haemoglobin and remove cells damaged by antibody is required if there is a positive Coombs test and the cord haemoglobin is below 12 g/dl (12 g/100ml) or the cord bilirubin is above 68 μmol/1 (4 mg/100 ml). A severely anaemic infant requires an urgent exchange transfusion. Cord haemoglobin levels may be erroneously low owing to the admixture of liquor or presence of a small clot in the specimen. These problems can be avoided by taking a second blood specimen with a wide bore needle from a large placental vein as soon as possible after the placenta has been delivered; the most satisfactory sample will be that with the higher haemoglobin level. In doubtful cases the haemoglobin should be repeated on a heel prick specimen before transfusion. The normal cord haemoglobin level is 14.5–20.5 g/dl (14.5–20.5 g/100 ml) and the normal heel prick haemoglobin level is 16–20 g/dl (16-20 g/100 ml). See p.89 for indications for later exchange transfusion.

DIABETES MELLITUS

There is a tendency for infants to be progressively heavier with each succeeding pregnancy and there is a danger of stillbirth towards term which is increased by poor control of the diabetes. If the diabetic control is poor, the infant's weight is above the 90th centile and he appears puffy and red and may develop hypoglycaemia or the respiratory distress syndrome (despite the weight) during the day after birth. In our experience hypoglycaemia can be prevented by continuous or frequent feeds of milk starting within 2 h after birth, and we consider that glucose feeds should be avoided; there is islet cell hyperplasia so that glucose may provoke an even more excessive secretion of insulin with consequent hypoglycaemia. Feeding is preceded by gastric lavage (see p.60). A Dextrostix test should be performed 3 hourly for the first 48 h of life followed by laboratory estimation of the blood glucose level if the Dextrostix test indicates that it is below 1.4 mmol/l (25 mg/100 ml). Asymptomatic hypoglycaemia is treated initially by feeding with milk and the Dextrostix test is repeated 1 h later (see p.83).

An apparently normal mother may have an infant with the features noted above. The infant is managed as though the mother had diabetes mellitus and the mother is investigated for prediabetes in the puerperium.

With the improved prognosis for infants of mothers with recognised diabetes mellitus, there has been increased attention to undiagnosed subclinical diabetes which is associated with a high perinatal mortality rate. It may be suspected in the antenatal period by the presence of persistent glycosuria in the second of the mother's fasting morning urine specimens and confirmed by a glucose tolerance test, preferably using the intravenous route. The possibility of subclinical diabetes should be considered if there is any family history of diabetes, a history of unexplained intrauterine death or of previous infants with birth weights over 4.5 kg.

INFECTION

Ruptured membranes over 24 h before delivery may lead to infected liquor and intrauterine pneumonia. Antibiotics given to the mother can cross the placenta.

Group B streptococci which are not normally considered to be dangerous pathogens in the mother can be virulent to the newborn infant and cause rapidly progressive septicaemia or pneumonia (see p.70).

Maternal urinary infection is associated with an increased incidence of urinary infection in the newborn infant. Herpes simplex virus (type 2) causes maternal vaginal and labial vesicular lesions which may infect the fetus by direct contact during vaginal delivery. Caesarean section is indicated to avoid neonatal herpes viraemia which is often fatal. If vaccination against smallpox is carried out during the early months of pregnancy the virus may pass the placenta causing generalised severe vaccinia in the fetus. No live virus vaccines should be given during pregnancy.

EXPOSURE TO DRUGS DURING PREGNANCY

Adverse effects on the fetus have been described when a mother has received one of over 40 different drugs. This suggests that *no* drug should be given in pregnancy unless there is a strong clinical indication. At the beginning of pregnancy, and preferably before conception, all the drugs prescribed should be reviewed to avoid unnecessary risk. Some drugs are essential to treat maternal disease but it may be possible to reduce the dose or substitute a safer alternative.

In proven urinary tract infection a 10-day course of ampicillin is given but prophylactic treatment for the rest of that pregnancy may be needed if there are several recurrences. Antibiotic sensitivities of the cultured bacteria will guide the choice of another drug if the pathogen is resistant to ampicillin. The preferred drugs include cephalexin, short-acting sulphonamides, e.g. sulphadimidine, or co-trimoxazole. Nitrofurantoin or nalidixic acid are safe but may cause vomiting. Although co-trimoxazole contains a folic acid antagonist and might be expected to cause fetal abnormalities, none have been reported despite the extensive use of this drug in pregnancy. A long-acting sulphonamide given to the mother passes to the fetus. If the infant is born shortly after a dose has been given, the drug may compete with bilirubin for binding sites on serum albumin with the result that the baby is at risk of developing kernicterus. Tetracycline may affect bone growth and induce staining of the infant's unerupted teeth.

Methyldopa is the most widely used drug for hypertension in pregnancy. Ganglion blocking agents may cause neonatal ileus. Frusemide is a safe diuretic, chlorothiazide may cause purpura in the infant. The penicillins are safe in pregnancy but streptomycin has been incriminated in some cases of congenital nerve deafness.

High doses of barbiturates or phenytoin in mothers with idiopathic epilepsy are associated with a higher than average incidence of cleft lip and other congenital abnormalities. The cause of this association is unknown but it may be possible to reduce the doses of the drugs if the maternal blood levels are above the therapeutic range.

Insulin provides the best diabetic control in pregnancy and avoids the possibility of congenital abnormalities and neonatal hypoglycaemia which might be caused by oral hypoglycaemic drugs.

High doses of steroids during pregnancy have been associated with fetal abnormalities in animals but there is no conclusive evidence that this occurs in man. Antithyroid drugs pass across the placenta and may induce transient hypothyroidism in the infant. Likewise iodides given to the mother in cough mixtures or in asthma powders may produce congenital goitre with hypothyroidism.

There is no completely satisfactory method of managing maternal venous thrombosis in pregnancy. Many units use warfarin until the 32nd week of gestation and in the puerperium. Heparin is given from 32 weeks until delivery. Warfarin given early in pregnancy has been associated with optic atrophy, mental retardation and bone changes in some infants.

Addiction to heroin in the mother may cause neonatal tremors, convulsions and death. Withdrawal symptoms have also been noted on rare occasions in babies born to mothers who have received large doses of barbiturates or other sedative drugs, but the more usual problem is general depression of the infant, especially respiratory centre depression. Recently diazepam has been used with success in the management of pre-eclamptic toxaemia but it may cause severe depression of the central control of respiration and temperature regulation. Diazepam is taken up by the tissues and later released so that the effects may be prolonged or recurrent for several days. The possible effects on the newborn infant of large doses of morphine or pethidine given to the mother during labour will be considered in Chapter 2 (see p.18).

Progestogens, for example norethisterone, given to the mother for threatened abortion may cause virilisation of the fetus. Norethisterone is no longer used as a test of pregnancy as it was associated with severe fetal anomalies. Cytotoxic drugs or moderate doses of radiation to the abdomen may cause fetal abnormalities. As the radiation hazard is confined to the early weeks of pregnancy, most radiologists insist that intravenous pyelograms and barium studies should be performed within the 9 days after a normal menstrual period.

A group of features including low birth weight, poor growth and mental retardation have been described in infants of mothers with chronic alcoholism and has been called the fetal alcohol syndrome. These mothers often have other high risk factors including smoking, malnutrition and social problems. The amount of alcohol needed and the timing of the effect are not known. Ideally attempts should be made to reduce the alcohol consumption before pregnancy begins.

CHAPTER TWO

Resuscitation of the Newborn

The 1970 British Birth Survey showed that 5% of infants did not establish respiration until more than 3 min after birth and 53% of the neonatal deaths were among this group.

Reasonable standards of care now demand that wherever babies are delivered there should be a person with adequate skill and experience in resuscitation immediately available throughout the 24 h. The paediatricians and anaesthetists are usually trained to provide this service and there should be no competitiveness in their roles. In some units it may be necessary for midwives or obstetric house surgeons to accept this responsibility, but it remains the paediatricians' and anaethetists' responsibility to ensure that effective training is given and the quality of care is monitored. Small units have the disadvantage that there are infrequent opportunities for intubation and inadequate supervision which may have disastrous consequences. Only in well-staffed, well-equipped, concentrated units can a completely satisfactory 24 h obstetric and paediatric service be maintained.

ASSESSMENT

In British hospitals about 7% of infants are intubated after birth. In about half these cases the need for intubation can be anticipated. The presence of a person skilled in intubation should be ensured in the following high risk situations — fetal distress, caesarean section, maternal anaesthetic, pre-term infant, breech delivery, difficult forceps delivery, twins, maternal diabetes and rhesus incompatibility. In a large proportion of infants who fail to breathe at birth none of these factors are present and for this reason a person capable of intubation must be immediately available throughout the 24 h.

The Apgar scoring system (see p.107) is still widely used as a method of assessing the infant's condition. The five items are usually scored at 1 min and 5 mins after birth. Ideally this score should be carried out by an assistant rather than the person in charge of resuscitation as active efforts to initiate breathing will be needed at 1 min if the infant is apnoeic at that time. There is a danger that in an effort to assess the Apgar score correctly, resuscitation will be delayed. As the heart rate and respiratory effort are the only items which determine the action to be taken, some units have abandoned the use of the Apgar score. Normal infants often can only obtain a maximum of 9 out of 10 points as the blue colour of the extremities is a normal finding.

RECOMMENDED INSTRUMENTS

1 Mucus extractor (Johnston and Johnston).
2 Appropriate small laryngoscope with short straight blade: 10 cm (spare battery and bulb for laryngoscope).
3 Endotracheal Cole type neonatal tubes (Portex) sizes FG8, 10, 12 (2, 2.5, 3 mm).
4 Suction catheters: (a) sizes FG6, 9, 14 (Portex PVC); (b) size FG4.5 (Argyle).
5 Intermittent positive pressure apparatus which can be provided by one of the following: (a) resuscitaire (Vickers); (b) anaesthetic bag and oxygen cylinder with pressure reducing valve and flow meter; (c) Penlon bag with endotracheal connection; (d) inflating bag and closely fitting face mask, e.g. Penlon or Ambu.
6 Soft rubber funnel for oxygen administration.

PROCEDURE

Immediately after delivery of the head, the infant's pharynx is aspirated by a mucus extractor with a fluid trap or a large-bore soft PVC catheter attached to a vacuum bottle. This procedure is carried out gently under direct vision and the catheter should not touch the back of the pharynx as reflex apnoea may occur. After complete delivery of the head, oxygen is given by funnel as long as central cyanosis is present (while the tongue is blue). If the infant does not breathe by 30 s after birth the closely fitting mask is applied to the face with the head extended, and the attached bag is squeezed a few times. If there are no respiratory movements at the end of 1 min after birth, or the heart rate is less than 100 per min at any time, the infant is placed supine on a flat surface.

The laryngoscope is held in the left hand and passed over the infant's tongue as far as the epiglottis (Fig.1(a),(b). The

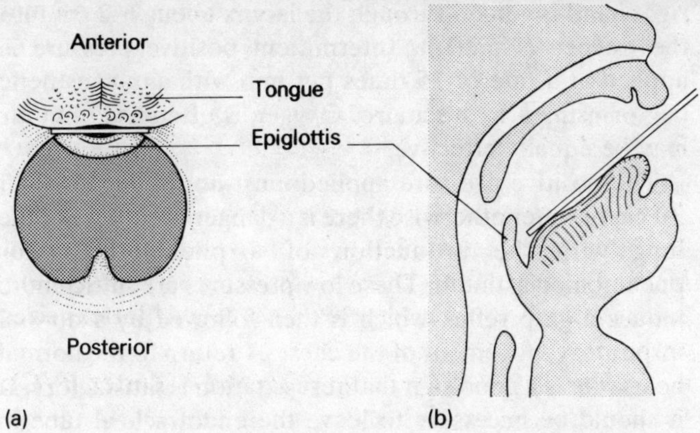

Fig. 1. Appearances during endotracheal intubation. (Modified from *The Lancet*, 1963, by kind permission of Dr H. Barrie and *The Lancet*.)

tip of the blade is advanced over the epiglottis about another 0.5 cm and is then withdrawn slightly. This presses the epiglottis against the root of the tongue revealing the glottis (Fig.2(a)). In the newborn the glottis is a slit in the centre of a small pink mound and the slit may expand into a triangular opening during a gasp. Gentle backward external pressure on the infant's larynx by an assistant may help to bring the glottis into view. Secretions are aspirated with a large catheter, e.g. FG9. The endotracheal tube held in the

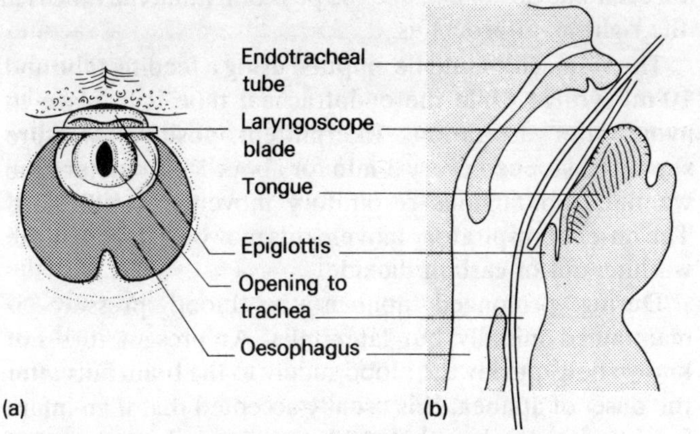

Fig. 2. Appearances during endotracheal intubation. (Modified from *The Lancet*, 1963, by kind permission of Dr. H. Barrie and *The Lancet*.)

right hand is guided through the larynx about 1–2 cm into the trachea (Fig.2(b)). Intermittent positive pressure is applied at a rate of 15 times per min with an anaesthetic bag or using a Resuscitaire. Oxygen is often used but air may be equally effective.

The positive pressure applied must not be higher than 30 cm of water otherwise there is a danger of rupture of the lung with the production of a pneumothorax or pneumomediastinum. These low pressures are sufficient to induce a gasp reflex which is then followed by a normal inspiratory movement of the chest. A return to the normal heart rate is a good sign that resuscitation is satisfactory. If it should be necessary to leave the endotracheal tube in place for a short period, the tube will be fixed to the cheek by adhesive tape.

Aspiration of secretions in the endotracheal tube can be carried out with a fine catheter (suction catheter FG4.5). The object of the shoulder on the Cole's tube and correct length of tube is to prevent the tube going into the right main bronchus but this may still occur. After introducing the endotracheal tube, it is advisable to check that it is in the trachea and not beyond the bifurcation of the trachea by noting that the chest movements and breath sounds heard with a stethoscope are equal on each side. This procedure is often recommended but normal breath sounds on each side do *not* exclude the possibility that the tube is in the right main bronchus.

The stomach should be emptied using a feeding tube and 10 ml syringe while the endotracheal tube is in place to avoid later aspiration. Intermittent positive pressure should be stopped every 3 min for about 15 s to determine whether spontaneous respiratory movements will start. The onset of respiratory movements may be delayed by the washing out of carbon dioxide.

During prolonged apnoea the blood pressure is maintained initially but later falls. At present it is not known how quickly the blood supply to the brain falls after the onset of apnoea. It is usually accepted that if an infant has a heart rate less than 100 per min, a short period of cardiac massage should be given at the same time as efforts to start respiratory movements. Cardiac massage can be carried out in the newborn by slight pressure with two fingers in the third and fourth intercostal spaces to the left of the sternum.

Hypothermia is a special hazard for infants who have been resuscitated and exposed during these procedures. Rapid initial drying of the infant with a warm towel is the most important preventive factor but resuscitation should also be carried out under a radiant heater of at least 400 W. It is important to realise that newborn infants are easily burned. The infant's rectal temperature should be checked with a low reading thermometer before the infant is transferred to the ward. Ideally a specially hot room at 30°C would be best for resuscitating pre-term infants, but this temperature is intolerable to mothers in labour and to staff. The infant should be wrapped up and handed to his mother for at least 1–2 min, even if he has later to be placed in a transport incubator and taken to the Special Care Unit. Most of the full term infants who have required resuscitation do *not* need to be admitted to the Special Care Unit.

FAILURE TO IMPROVE

The best sign that resuscitation is successful is the increase in heart rate. If this does not occur within about 15 s the following should be considered:

1 The gas cylinders may be empty or the pipeline disconnected.

2 The endotracheal tube may have been misplaced into the oesophagus or have slipped out of the trachea during extension of the neck. If there are breath sounds of equal intensity on each side of the chest this possibility is unlikely. If there is any doubt the endotracheal tube should be removed and a fresh tube inserted immediately.

3 The endotracheal tube may have been placed too far down so that only the right main bronchus is being inflated. In this case there will be unequal breath sounds on each side of the chest.

After these possibilities have been excluded the most common possibilities are pulmonary hypoplasia or diaphragmatic hernia. Pulmonary hypoplasia accompanies renal abnormalities in Potter's syndrome. In this condition oligohydramnios is often found during pregnancy and the infant's face appears compressed with furrows on the forehead. The ears are large, lack cartilage and are low set. These infants are usually stillborn or die within a few hours of birth. In diaphragmatic hernia the abdominal viscera compress the lung and as the lesion is usually left-sided there is apparent dextrocardia. Immediate chest X-ray is necessary for diagnosis and both an endotracheal tube and gastric tube should remain in place until the infant reaches the operating theatre.

DRUGS

If the mother has received pethidine or morphine, a chemical antagonist can be given to the infant. Alternatively it can be given to the mother by the intravenous route before delivery.

If the infant needs intubation and drugs, intubation is performed first. Naloxone is given preferably intramuscularly in a dose of 0.02 mg/kg body weight. Higher doses up to a total of 0.2 mg have been recommended but this is still under trial. There is no advantage in giving drugs intravenously via the umbilical vein when endotracheal intubation is carried out, since the baby's respiration will be supported until an intramuscular dose has had time to take effect. The temptation to administer drugs via the umbilical vein is great but it is not without risk, and the authors deprecate the frequent unnecessary use of this route. Naloxone does not cause respiratory depression itself but its main disadvantage is the short period of action. If given intravenously high plasma levels are present for about 30 min and when given intramuscularly from 30 min to 24 h after the dose. It may therefore be necessary to repeat the dose of naloxone if the intravenous route is used alone as the effects of the pethidine may be present for many hours.

If the heart rate has been very low and cardiac massage has been necessary, the possibility of giving intravenous glucose and alkali should be considered. It must be emphasised that an adequate supply of oxygen quickly reverses acidosis and this is the best and safest means in most infants. It should also be noted that 8.4% sodium bicarbonate solution is extremely hypertonic and 1 part must be diluted with 5 parts of sterile water to produce an isotonic solution. In the severely asphyxiated infant it is reasonable to give 1 mmol/kg body weight of sodium bicarbonate which is 1 ml/kg of an 8.4% solution diluted in sterile water at a rate of 1–2 ml/min using an umbilical vein catheter.

WHEN NOT TO INTUBATE

If the infant is less than 26 weeks gestation as shown by fused eyelids, resuscitation should not be attempted. Anencephaly is another contraindication. Infants with Down's syndrome or myelomeningocoele are difficult problems and the decision cannot be made by a member of the junior staff. Prior consultation with a consultant may be possible but otherwise it is best to resuscitate and reconsider the question later. If the heart rate has been recorded at any time during the second stage of labour, resuscitation should be attempted even if there is no heart beat at birth. If no heart beat is obtained 20 min after beginning resuscitation, the attempt should be abandoned. If the heart rate is normal but the infant is not breathing spontaneously half an hour after starting resuscitation, the problem should be discussed with a consultant if he is immediately available, or alternatively the infant should be placed on a ventilator and the decision made later.

DISCUSSION WITH PARENTS

If the infant is breathing normally without delay he should be given to his mother after a rapid examination. It should be mentioned that the child appears to be normal and that it is common for infants to need help with breathing at birth. It is important to stress that his progress will be no different from that of other infants who have not needed resuscitation. The majority of infants who have required intubation should go with their mothers to the postnatal wards and receive routine observations. Only if there has been a prolonged period before spontaneous respiration has been established, should the infant be taken to the Special Care Unit. If resuscitation has not been successful, the person responsible for resuscitation, together with a member of the obstetric staff, should see both parents immediately. The parents should be asked whether they would like to see the dead infant, who should be suitably wrapped up before being brought in to them. It is usual for a member of the nursing staff to be with the parents and she can answer questions about the baby's appearance. It may become apparent that the mother is anxious to hold the baby and if so, it may be kinder to leave her alone to grieve over her dead baby for a few minutes. Discussion with the parents will help to decide who is the best person to help them with their grieving and with the reactions of the other children in the family. The family doctor should be informed by telephone as soon as possible.

These recommendations apply equally when there has been a delivery of a stillborn infant. Failing to grieve has been the starting point for depressive illness in some instances.

CHAPTER THREE

Routine Examination of the Newborn

Immediately after birth all infants are examined for the presence of gross congenital abnormalities or evidence of birth trauma. (The most common abnormalities are noted in the next chapter.) Later, every infant should be examined again in detail by the paediatric house physician or obstetric house surgeon. This chapter is concerned with the detailed routine examination.

It is best to perform this examination on the morning after delivery as this avoids missing patients who are going to be discharged home at 48 h. The mother should be present as this gives her an opportunity to express her anxieties, and for the results of the examination to be discussed with her. The obstetric notes should be perused to check the expected date of delivery and to determine whether the infant has been at special risk, e.g. maternal rubella or a difficult delivery. A systematic approach should be used in order to save time and avoid missing abnormalities. If any abnormality is found, a nurse should be present while the mother is being informed. The examination need not take a long time if the mother or a nurse is present to undress and dress the infant. Even if no abnormalities are found, the results of the examination should be recorded in the notes.

HISTORY

Maternal and obstetric

Light-for-dates and large-for-dates infants are liable to hypoglycaemia (see p.81).

Polyhydramnios is associated with a high incidence of fetal abnormalities, especially anencephaly and oesophageal atresia. Infants born before arrival at hospital are liable to have sustained an injury or may be hypothermic. A single umbilical artery is frequently associated with other congenital abnormalities, particularly renal. The umbilical arteries can be recognised in the freshly cut cord as two slightly protruding thick walled vessels which do not gape. It is convenient to check that both arteries are present by cutting the cord again when examining the placenta.

If the placenta is less than one-sixth of the infant's weight or infarction is present, the possibility of intrauterine malnutrition and liability to neonatal hypoglycaemia should be considered.

Family

The family history may raise a suspicion of cystic fibrosis, congenital dislocation of the hip, adrenogenital syndrome or other inherited disorders.

PHYSICAL EXAMINATION

The infant must be completely undressed and in a good light.

General observation

1 Pallor may be due to severe anaemia caused by slipping of a ligature from the umbilical cord, cephalhaematoma, haemorrhagic disease of the newborn or, rarely, rupture of the liver or transfer of blood from one twin into the other. Bleeding from an umbilical vessel perforated during amniocentesis may cause severe anaemia. An urgent blood transfusion may be necessary.
2 Jaundice appearing within 24 h of birth is likely to be due to haemolytic disease.
3 Diffuse capillary naevi on the face, eyelids or occiput are common.

The 'strawberry mark' starts as a tiny red spot and grows rapidly over several weeks until it has a raised red appearance with small white areas suggesting the 'seeds' of a strawberry. These are more common in pre-term babies. They may occur anywhere on the body but do not cause symptoms except on the eyelids where they cause difficulty in opening the eyes and require treatment. Strawberry naevi increase in size, often rapidly for 3–9 months. At least 90% of these naevi undergo complete or partial spontaneous resolution which commonly begins between the ages of 6 and 12 months and is usually complete in 50% by the age of 5, and in 70% by 7 years. These naevi will resolve completely without trace in over 80% of cases.

The port wine stain is not raised and may be extensive. Unfortunately it shows no tendency to resolve but the skin texture remains normal. When the naevus occurs in the distribution of the trigeminal nerve, there is a possibility of an associated intracranial vascular anomaly.

4 Purpura. When this is present only on the head it may be due to pressure on the neck during delivery or pressure on the face due to face presentation. Although commonly found after the cord has compressed the neck it also follows many apparently normal vertex deliveries. Subconjunctival haemorrhages have a similar significance.

When purpura is generalised it is usually due to deficiency of platelets, the cause of which requires investigation.

5 Cyanosis of the hands and feet with a normally coloured tongue has no pathological significance.

6 Neonatal urticaria (erythema toxicum). Blotchy ill-defined areas of bright erythema surround white or yellow wheals which resemble septic spots. Neonatal urticaria usually appears on the 2nd day of life and in most infants clears within 48 h. The lesions contain many eosinophils and have no pathological significance. By ringing individual lesions with a skin pencil it can be shown that they disappear in a few hours to be replaced by others elsewhere. This contrasts with septic lesions which appear later and do not resolve so quickly (see p.99).

7 Mongolian blue spots are patchy accumulations of pigment especially over the buttocks and lower back in infants of races in whom pigmentation of the skin occurs. They are common in babies of African or Mongolian descent, but also occur in other babies, e.g. Italian or Greek. They may be mistaken for bruises and an erroneous diagnosis of battered baby syndrome made. They become less obvious as the rest of the skin darkens.

8 Polycythaemia is a packed cell volume exceeding 70%. This syndrome may occur in one of identical twins who has received blood from the other twin through a placental vascular connection. Polycythaemia may also occur following delayed clamping of the cord or in infants of diabetic mothers. Symptoms ascribed to polycythaemia have included fits, congestive cardiac failure, respiratory distress or severe jaundice. If polycythaemia is causing significant symptoms a partial exchange transfusion can be performed with 0.9% sodium chloride solution using 20 ml/kg.

9 The Harlequin colour change is unilateral redness stopping abruptly at the midline. It may occur during the first few days in normal infants as a transient phenomenon. It affects the side on which the baby is lying, suggesting that gravity is a causative factor.

10 Accessory nipples have no pathological significance. Typically they resemble a miniature nipple and may be present in the midclavicular line between the clavicles and groins: sometimes there is no more than a tiny pigmented spot.

11 Congenital glaucoma should be suspected if there is clouding of the cornea or the eye appears excessively large. Urgent advice from the opthalmologist will be needed.

12 The most common site for a midline pit over the spine is over the coccyx but this type does not communicate with the spinal canal. A midline pit anywhere else along the spine may be connected with an underlying sinus which may communicate with the spinal canal and requires excision to prevent the entry of bacteria and subsequent meningitis.

Head and neck

1 Oesophageal atresia with or without tracheo-oesophageal fistula. Frothy mucus dribbles persistently from the mouth. --- secretions/saliva - not swallowed

2 Pierre Robin syndrome. Small lower jaw, glossoptosis and cleft palate. The infant must be nursed prone to avoid the tongue falling backwards and occluding the airway. A small jaw (micrognathia) may occur alone or with other abnormalities.

3 Nodules of epithelial cells resembling pearls (Epstein's pearls) just lateral to the midline on the hard palate are a normal finding. A cluster of these pearls is present at the junction of the hard and soft palates.

4 Potter facies. Characterised especially by the presence of large, poorly cartilaginised, low set ears. It accompanies bilateral renal agenesis or other severe abnormality of the kidneys, often with pulmonary hypoplasia.

Cardiovascular system

The apex beat is palpated but it may be difficult to detect in the newborn. Palpation below the xyphisternum will show whether there is excessive pulsation as an indication of cardiac enlargement. If the femoral pulses are weak or absent, coarctation of the aorta or hypoplastic left heart syndrome should be considered. The blood pressure is taken with a Doppler ultrasonic flowmeter in all four limbs and low pressures in the lower limbs confirm the diagnosis of narrowing of the aorta below the origin of the ductus arteriosus. If the lesion is above this level there may be no difference between the pressures in the arms and legs. Typically, patent ductus arteriosus produces a continuous murmur but the murmur is often systolic at this stage and this may lead to difficulties in diagnosis. Often there is a large pulse pressure which makes the dorsalis pedis pulse easily palpable. Soft basal murmurs come and go in the normal newborn infant but harsh basal murmurs are likely to be due to aortic or pulmonary stenosis.

The commonest form of congenital heart disease, ventricular septal defect, does not produce symptoms until about 3 weeks after birth and there may be no murmur until that time; but with careful auscultation a systolic murmur is usually audible towards the end of the 1st week of life. If a significant murmur is heard during the routine examination in the first 24h of life, it is likely to be due to a patent ductus arteriosus or stenosis of the aortic or pulmonary valves. We have found a plan helpful in management of an infant with a systolic murmur found at a routine examination (see next page). Heart failure in the 1st week of life is usually due to multiple defects especially transposition of the great arteries or hypoplastic left heart syndrome. Occasionally persistence of some of the fetal circulatory haemodynamics after birth causes transient heart failure. Any infant with cyanotic congenital heart disease or heart failure should be given digoxin and sent to a specialised unit without delay. Infants who are *not* cyanosed should be given frusemide as well as digoxin.

MURMUR HEARD DURING FIRST 2 DAYS OF LIFE

Short systolic murmur in an infant who is feeding well

Palpate all pulses. Do *not* perform ECG or chest X-ray. If the infant can be examined again on the 7th day, do not mention the murmur to the mother. Otherwise tell the mother, or preferably both parents, that you have heard a soft noise in the chest which will probably disappear by itself. Arrange for the infant to be seen in the Outpatient clinic when 3 weeks old. Inform family doctor.

Loud, long systolic murmur, or an infant who is feeding poorly

Palpate all pulses. Arrange for an ECG and chest X-ray to be carried out the same day and ensure that the baby is seen by a paediatrician without delay.

MURMUR HEARD AROUND 8TH DAY

Chest X-ray and ECG should be performed and the infant seen by a paediatrician. The majority of these murmurs are due to a ventricular septal defect or mild pulmonary stenosis. Most of the ventricular septal defects close spontaneously before the infants are 5 years of age.

Respiratory system

The normal respiratory rate at rest is below 50/min and there should be no recession of the chest wall or under the mandible.

Abdomen

GENERAL

The umbilicus is inspected for signs of infection. Normally the liver is easily palpable, the edge being about 2 cm below the right costal margin in the midclavicular line. A large bladder after micturition suggests urethral obstruction. The anus should be examined for patency and position.

GENITALIA

A hooded prepuce suggests hypospadias with the urethral orifice at the base of the glans penis. If the urinary meatus is adequate and there is no curvature of the penis (chordee), no immediate treatment is required. Circumcision must *not* be performed and the infant should be referred to the next clinic of the plastic surgeon.

If the urethral orifice is nearer the perineum, adrenogenital syndrome should be considered. In the adrenogenital syndrome there is failure to secrete cortisol with excessive androgen production by the adrenals. Female infants become virilised with enlargement of the clitoris and fusion of the labia, and may be mistaken for males. In males the genitalia are normal.

A less common cause of ambiguity of the external genitalia is intersex. Chromosomal or hormonal factors may be involved. A paediatrician should be consulted without delay if an infant has ambiguity of the genitalia in view of the serious social implications.

Small hydrocoeles usually disappear spontaneously during the 1st month.

Undescended testis is especially common in pre-term infants in whom the testes usually descend during the first 3 months after birth. A full term infant with failure of descent of one or both testis should be referred for a surgical opinion. As the cremasteric reflex is usually absent at birth, the testis cannot be retractile. The scrotum is poorly developed on the side of the undescended testis. If there is doubt whether a testis is descended the following procedure for the examination is recommended.

1 Palpate pubic tubercle with one hand.

2 Hold testis between thumb and forefinger of the other hand, gently draw down to its fullest extent.

3 Measure from pubic tubercle to centre of firm globular testis.

4 At term the testis, if fully descended, lies between 4 and 7 cm from the tubercle.
5 If the measured distance is less than 4 cm in full term infants the testis has not descended.
6 In pre-term infants who are more likely to have undescended testes and whose testes are smaller, 2.5 cm has been arbitrarily chosen to divide descent from non-descent.

A small amount of vaginal bleeding is common and follows the excretion of maternal or placental oestrogens which were transmitted to the fetus before birth. It is commonly observed 5–7 days after birth. A white vaginal discharge or prolapse of the vaginal mucosa are normal.

STOOLS

Meconium, which is sticky, greenish-black material is passed up to 48 h; 'changing stools' which are greenish-brown with some milk curds for a further 3 days; and then normal 'milk' stools are passed. Sometimes a white plug is passed before the first meconium. Prolonged delay in passage of meconium could indicate the presence of intestinal obstruction.

URINE

Urine is usually passed within a few hours of birth. Rarely, and probably due to the passage of urine during delivery, no further urine may be passed for 36 h in a normal infant. After this time, the possibility of a urethal valve in the male should be considered, and can be excluded if there is a good stream when urine is passed. Dehydration and oliguria may be due to intestinal obstruction. The first urine often contains urates which appear red on the napkin and resemble blood.

Limbs

1 Congenital dislocated hip and dislocatable hip. This is the most important asymptomatic congenital abnormality to detect as treatment is extremely effective. The total incidence of dislocated and dislocatable hip in the first 2 days of life is about 1 in 100 live births. If these are not treated, the incidence of established dislocated hip is 1 in 800 live births. The anomaly is more common in girls, especially after breech delivery, and there is a high incidence in some families. There is also racial predisposition, the condition being more common in Italians. Recognition requires adequate training and practice, and the following method is recommended.

The hands are warmed and the infant approached gently as muscular relaxation is essential for a reliable examination. The infant may be induced to be more relaxed by putting a teat in her mouth. With the infant on her back the degree of abduction of the femora at rest is noted. The

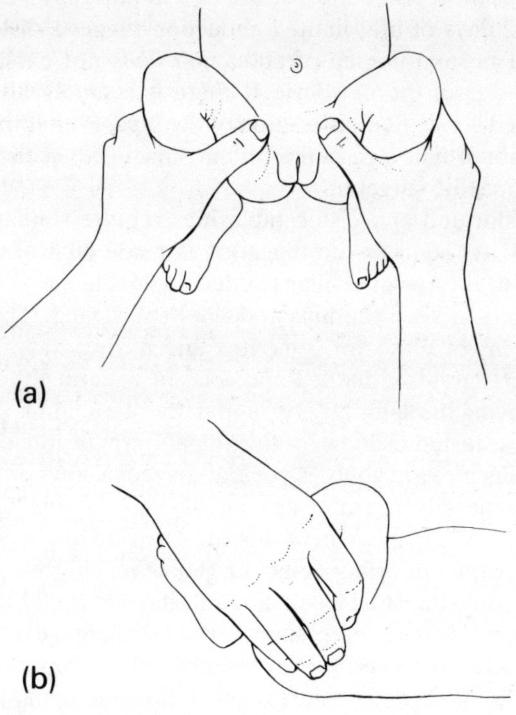

Fig. 3.

knees and hips are flexed to a right angle and the greater trochanter is grasped between the examiner's thumb anteriorly and his fingers posteriorly (Fig.3(a),(b)). Each leg is held in slight abduction. Holding the knees alone must be avoided, as this produces dangerous leverage. An attempt is made to move each femoral head gently forwards into or backwards out of the acetabulum. Results fall into one of three groups: (a) no movement of femoral head—normal hip; (b) femoral head moves forwards—dislocated hip. (c) femoral head moves backwards—dislocatable hip.

Movement of the femoral head in and out of the acetabulum is the only reliable sign. It may be accompanied by a peculiar 'clonking' sensation but this must be distinguished from a ligamentous click which has no pathological significance. Abduction of the hips is normally 90° in the first 2 days of life; limited abduction suggests dislocation but a normal degree of abduction does not exclude the diagnosis in the newborn. If there is a family history of treated congenital dislocation of the hips, even if there are no abnormal signs, the infant must be seen by an orthopaedic surgeon.

Dislocated and dislocatable hips require similar treatment. As soon as the diagnosis is made clinically a von Rosen, Barlow or similar padded malleable metal splint is applied to keep the hips abducted and flexed. The splint remains in place for 3 months and during this time the infant should be bathed and washed without the mother removing the splint. It is essential that the splint is periodically adjusted to allow for the infant's growth and to ensure that the hips are not being overabducted. X-rays of the hips are generally not of value in diagnosis in the neonatal period. The management should be carried out in conjunction with an orthopaedic surgeon. When the splint is removed almost all treated infants have normal hips. Late diagnosis leads to permanent secondary damage to the hips and often the need for several orthopaedic operations.

This management and prognosis does not apply to dislocation related to other congenital abnormalities, e.g. myelomeningocoele.

2 Talipes (club foot). The commonest reason for an abnormal shape of the feet is muscular imbalance due to the posture of the feet of the infant while in utero. In postural talipes it should be possible to dorsiflex the foot fully and to obtain passive inversion to 90° and eversion to 60°. The mother can be taught to manipulate the foot through the whole range of movements after each feed, although it will usually revert to normal within a few weeks even without treatment but it may persist in a mild degree for several months. In contrast, in structural talipes the range of passive movements is restricted and orthopaedic advice regarding strapping, manipulation or serial plasters is needed within 24 h.

3 Extra digits. The digits should be counted with the palms open otherwise an extra thumb may be missed. Polydactyly requires the advice of a plastic surgeon to determine which digit should be removed for the best functional result. Extra fingers and toes are often familial and vary from an apparently normal digit to a skin tag. The latter can be tied off with a linen thread and will separate by aseptic necrosis.

Central nervous system

Alertness and the symmetry of spontaneous movements are noted. The anterior fontanelle tension and width of the fontanelle are palpated while the infant is at rest and the head circumference is measured. A more detailed neurological examination is *not* required unless there is a special indication.

Biochemistry

GUTHRIE TEST

Drops of blood taken by heel prick after 6 days of breast or bottle milk feeding (usually 7th day of life) are placed on the special absorbent card provided. The blood is examined for the presence of a high level of phenylalanine found in patients with phenylketonuria. Some of these babies need a special diet to prevent brain damage.

TALKING TO PARENTS

If possible both parents should be seen together. If an abnormality is found during a routine examination, some indication must be given to the mother so that arrangements can be made to see both parents. Particularly if the problem is likely to be a longterm one, a senior member of the paediatric staff who is likely to continue the longterm care should speak to the parents initially. If a junior member of the staff has had limited experience of a particular problem, it is better to tell the parents that he needs to seek further advice rather than guess at the answer. Parents often cling to the first opinion and may find it difficult to accept the more experienced views later. It is possible to give a statement of the facts, for example that there is an abnormality of the spine, with the assurance that a more senior member of the staff will discuss the problem within a short period. A member of the nursing staff should always be present, as she is likely to be asked all the questions again as soon as the doctor has left. Ideally the interview should take place in a quiet room without telephone or bleeps, with adequate time.

The diagnosis should be explained in terms the parents can understand, although it may only be presumptive. For example, if the probable diagnosis is ventricular septal defect, it is not necessary to explain that there is a remote possibility of multiple cardiac defects. In discussing management, the help and support that will be given by social workers or physiotherapists should be stressed from the beginning and the parents should be advised to tell their relations and friends the diagnosis rather than hide it. In considering prognosis, the positive aspects should be stressed with as much optimism as possible. For example, after a difficult forceps delivery it is better to indicate that most such babies will develop normally rather than say they may be slightly backward. Unnecessarily pessimistic prognosis based on out-of-date information can alter a mother's attitude to her baby and impair maternal infant attachment.

CHAPTER FOUR

Congenital Abnormalities

CENTRAL NERVOUS SYSTEM

Myelomeningocoele

There is a flat or raised neural plaque in the midline over the spine due to abnormal development of the spinal cord associated with deficiency of the dorsal laminae and dorsal spines of the vertebrae. It is most commonly found in the lumbar region. The associated absence of the various coverings which normally protect the cord allows meningitis to occur easily. If there are no active movements in the legs and the anus is patulous it is very likely that the infant will be incontinent of urine and faeces and will never be able to walk unaided. Thoracic lesions and kyphosis are signs of poor prognosis. The sensory level, which can be tested with an opened paper clip, is usually similar to the motor defect level. Hydrocephalus at birth, as shown by a head circumference more than 2 cm above that expected for the weight centile, indicates a poor outlook. In view of the need for urgent treatment for those with a good prognosis, it is advised that all affected infants should either be seen by a consultant paediatrician without delay, or sent to a special centre where selection for surgery can be made.

The majority of these infants develop progressive hydrocephalus later and those considered suitable for surgery require insertion of a catheter, with a valve, from the brain to the lower end of the superior vena cava in order to reduce the cerebrospinal fluid pressure. Progressive hydrocephalus is confirmed by measuring the circumference of the head at its largest diameter (occipitofrontal) every 3 days with a disposal paper tape measure, plotting these values on a special chart, and showing that the head is growing at a faster rate than normal (see p.109). A comparable anomaly of the brain, usually in the occipital region, is known as an encephalocoele.

Anencephaly

Absence of cranial vault and most of the brain. The diagnosis is obvious on gross inspection and the infant dies during or shortly after birth (see p.124).

Microcephaly

This is a small head which is especially noticed by the forehead appearing small in relation to the face. Diagnosis is confirmed by demonstrating a small occipitofrontal circumference in relation to the baby's weight and gestational age. It is invariably associated with mental impairment. It can be due to infection during pregnancy, e.g. rubella, cytomegalovirus or toxoplasmosis and a sample of the mother's blood should be screened for these infections. In the infant the presence of specific IgM to one of these infections confirms fetal infection, but rarely may be absent at the initial examination and should be estimated again after 6 months. A knowledge of the probable aetiology would help in genetic counselling.

CLEFT LIP AND CLEFT PALATE

These abnormalities are frequently associated. A cleft lip may be unilateral or bilateral and is due to failure of the maxillary process growing towards the midline to fuse with the premaxilla. The rare central cleft lip is associated with some cerebral malformation.. Minor degrees of cleft palate can be easily missed if the hard palate is not seen and palpated. A bifid uvula may indicate a muscular defect with a mucosal covering; mobility of the soft palate is impaired so that symptoms may be identical to those which occur when the cleft is complete, namely regurgitation of feeds through the nose and difficulty with speech.

The lip should be repaired at 3 months and the palate at 1 year. If there are feeding difficulties, a special teat, a large normal teat, a special spade-like spoon or an ordinary spoon may be tried. The value of an obturator before operative closure is controversial.

ABDOMINAL WALL

Omphalocoele

This is a hernia into the base of the umbilical cord and contains gut and sometimes solid organs like the liver. In contrast to a true umbilical hernia the sac is covered by peritoneum but no skin. Immediate surgical repair is usually required although in some centres large lesions have been successfully treated with a silastic bag or repeated local applications of a sclerosing fluid such as 2% aqueous Merthiolate.

Umbilical hernia

This is a hernia at the umbilicus usually containing omentum and gut which is most common in African infants or West Indians of African descent. No treatment is required as the hernia usually disappears spontaneously by the age of 3 years, although in West Indian infants it may take a further 3 years.

'Prune belly' syndrome

Absence of abdominal muscles causes a puckered appearance of the abdominal wall. It usually occurs in males and is almost always associated with dilatation of the entire urinary tract and cryptorchidism.

RENAL TRACT

Polycystic kidneys

Enlarged kidneys may be due to polycystic disease which may be familial.

Ectopia vesicae (exstrophy of the bladder)

Failure of development of the anterior wall of the bladder and the lower abdominal wall leaves the posterior wall of the bladder and ureteric openings exposed. The medial portions of the pubic bones are deficient and the ends must be approximated before plastic surgery can be performed. The upper renal tract may or may not be normal and ascending infection is less common than might be expected.

Posterior urethral valve

This is the commonest form of lower urinary tract obstruction in boys. The presenting feature may be a poor urinary stream, abdominal distension from an enlarged bladder, urinary tract infection, or rarely urinary ascites following a leak from the urinary tract. Bilateral nephrostomy and later removal of the valve is required. Severe renal damage may be present at birth due to back pressure during intrauterine life.

ALIMENTARY TRACT

Oesophageal atresia

It is a common practice in many units to pass a tube into the stomach as part of the initial examination to exclude oesophageal atresia. In the absence of such a routine diagnostic manœuvre, the diagnosis will be suspected in any baby in whom there is continual accumulation of frothy secretions in the mouth and sometimes with cyanotic attacks.

The first feed should be supervised by the most experienced nurse on the ward. In many units 5% glucose solution is given as the first feed to reduce the dangers of aspiration pneumonia if oesophageal atresia and tracheo-oesophageal fistula are present. The diagnosis of oesophageal atresia is confirmed by attempting to pass a tube down the oesophagus. The tube used must be sufficiently stiff to prevent coiling in the upper oesophageal pouch and should have a radio-opaque tip. We have found a FG9 feeding tube with a radio-opaque thread can be used. If the passage of the tube is impeded, a chest X-ray is taken with the tube *gently* pushed down as far as it will go to check the site of the obstruction. When the lower part of the oesophagus has a fistulous connection with the trachea (indicated by the presence of gas in the stomach and intestines) this is usually about 1 cm above the carina. The use of radio-opaque fluids is not necessary and has obvious disadvantages.

Ano-rectal malformation

The anus is examined for patency and position.

Intestinal obstruction (see p.59).

LIMBS (see previous chapter).

MULTIPLE ABNORMALITIES

Trisomy 21 (Mongolism—Down's syndrome)

The palpebral fissures slant upwards and outwards, prominent epicanthic folds, occiput flat, single palmar crease, distal palmar triradius, poor limb tone, congenital heart disease, severe mental retardation.

Trisomy 18 (Edward's syndrome)

Intrauterine and postnatal failure to thrive. Low set deformed ears, small mandible, flexion deformity of fingers, prominent heels, congenital heart disease, mental retardation.

Trisomy 13 (Patau's syndrome)

Cleft lip and palate, microphthalmia, large nose, prominent heels, polydactyly, congenital heart and renal disease, mental retardation.

Turner's syndrome (X0)

Webbing of neck or loose skin folds at the back of the neck, low posterior hairline, broad chest with widely spaced nipples, renal and cardiac defects especially coarctation of the aorta. Oedema of the hands and feet, which does not usually pit, is often prominent in the neonatal period, and is a useful diagnostic feature.

Rubella syndrome

Deafness, congenital heart disease (especially patent ductus arteriosus), cataract, thrombocytopenic purpura, hepatitis, retinitis, encephalitis, X-ray changes at metaphyses of long bones, and rarely glaucoma.

Cytomegalovirus infection

Hepatosplenomegaly, jaundice, purpura, chorioretinitis, microcephaly, cerebral calcification radiologically.

Toxoplasmosis

Chorioretinitis, convulsions, hydrocephalus, intracranial calcification radiologically, jaundice, hepatosplenomegaly, lymphadenopathy, rash, anaemia.

Mental retardation cannot be assessed accurately in the neonatal period but has been included for prognosis. Every patient with a particular syndrome does not have all the features listed.

CHROMOSOME STUDIES

Chromosome studies are used to confirm the diagnosis or to clarify the diagnosis when the clinical features are atypical. Chromosome studies using peripheral lymphocyte culture can produce results in a few days but results from bone marrow aspirated from the tibia are available in a few hours if an answer is needed urgently; for example, in an infant with mongolism and duodenal atresia.

CHAPTER FIVE

Birth Trauma

HEAD

Intracranial

Although it is not usually thought of as a form of injury it should be noted that anoxia is the commonest cause of 'cerebral' signs. Premature separation of the placenta, placental infarction, or the cord tightly round the neck predispose to anoxia which may be followed by petechial, subarachnoid and intracerebral haemorrhages.

Intraventricular and subarachnoid haemorrhages are found in pre-term infants and are a common cause of death in infants with the respiratory distress syndrome.

When the fetal head is large in relation to the pelvic outlet, or delivery is precipitate or by the breech there is a risk of extracerebral haemorrhage due to laceration of the tentorium cerebelli or falx cerebri involving a venous sinus.

Infants may be unduly lethargic or especially irritable shortly after birth, but there are usually no helpful confirmatory signs at this stage. Later there may be pallor, high pitched cry, poor muscle tone or increased tone, convulsions, reluctance to suck, vomiting, apnoeic attacks, and fast or periodic breathing. Rarely the heart rate is slow, the pupils are unequal and fail to react to light or the anterior fontanelle tension is raised. A Dextrostix test should be performed to exclude hypoglycaemia and a lumbar puncture should be considered to exclude meningitis.

The infant is nursed in an incubator to facilitate observation but if the baby weighs over 3 kg the thermostat is turned to the minimum level.

If convulsions occur the following method of management has been found to be successful. An intramuscular injection of paraldehyde is given. The addition of hyaluronidase made up with water and well shaken accelerates the onset of the maximum therapeutic effect of paraldehyde by increasing the rate of absorption.

Afterwards an intravenous infusion is started. About 2 h after the fit has occurred phenytoin 8 mg/kg is given intravenously over 15 min to prevent a recurrence. Twenty-four hours later the maintenance dose of phenytoin is started but can usually be discontinued after 48 h. Alternatively intramuscular phenobarbitone can be given instead of phenytoin. Doubts have been cast on using phenytoin in the 1st year of life, as there is evidence that it may interfere with cerebellar maturation which occurs at this time. However this is not a serious contraindication to short-term use of the drug and it has the great advantage that it does not lower the level of consciousness or make the infant reluctant to suck. Oral feeds are stopped for 24 h and fluids are given intravenously.

The respiratory distress syndrome may cause cerebral anoxia and the cerebral signs may predominate.

Cephalhaematoma

This is a subperiosteal haemorrhage which is limited by the surrounding sutures. It is believed that in the majority there is a hairline fracture of the underlying cranial bone which may be difficult to demonstrate, but is unimportant as it involves only the outer table. There is usually no brain damage. A surprisingly large amount of blood may be present and a blood transfusion is occasionally required. The lesion may not be noticed until the 3rd day. During subsequent resolution a calcified rim may appear which suggests a depressed fracture or there may be a hard swelling which takes several months to disappear. Cephalhaematoma must be distinguished from caput succedaneum which is a soft tissue swelling due to oedema of the part of the head presenting at the cervix and it is not limited by the sutures.

'Chignon'

Vacuum extraction is often associated with a 'chignon' or subcutaneous oedema where the cap has been applied. In some instances this may become a large haematoma and occasionally the skin becomes necrotic. However, the skin grows rapidly from the borders to cover the area within a few weeks. It must be distinguished from congenital absence of skin of the scalp when it occurs in the midline since these lesions are sometimes associated with underlying bone defects.

Fractures of the skull

Linear fractures are usually associated with severe cerebral injury but often pass undetected because it is the cerebral injury which is the cause of the symptoms. Depressed fractures are usually quite benign, but elevation of the fracture should be considered if there is evidence of underlying brain damage, or, later, for cosmetic reasons.

Facial palsy

Direct pressure by obstetric forceps on the facial nerve may cause a transient palsy which lasts up to 2 weeks. Often there is an area of fat necrosis to confirm the traumatic aetiology (see below)). Care of the exposed cornea is essential.

SHOULDER

1 Fracture of clavicle.
2 Fracture of humerus.
3 Stretching of brachial plexus

These present as lack of spontaneous movements and absent Moro reflex in the appropriate arm. The clavicle and humerus should be X-rayed. Fracture of the clavicle requires no treatment and for fracture of the humerus the arm is splinted to the infant's chest by a crêpe bandage. Injuries to the brachial plexus occasionally have a poor prognosis and the infant should be seen by an orthopaedic surgeon for advice on the prevention of contractures. Diaphragmatic paralysis often accompanies stretching of the brachial plexus and may cause a raised respiratory rate.

Pressure on the radial nerve in the radial groove causes temporary paralysis of the dorsiflexors of the wrist, which may be mistaken for a brachial plexus injury. The diagnosis is confirmed by finding an area of fat necrosis on the posterolateral aspect of the upper arm.

STERNOMASTOID 'TUMOUR'

This is not noticeable at birth but usually presents after the 1st week. The firm mass 1–2 cm in diameter may be situated anywhere along the length of the sternomastoid muscle, but is usually in the middle or lower third. It may be due to a small haematoma or fibromatous malformation. They all disappear within the 1st year. Torticollis is sometimes present. This is because the congenitally short sternomastoid muscle associated with torticollis is particularly prone to the injury which causes a sternomastoid tumour. If sternomastoid tumour ever causes torticollis it is noticed much later (at about 5 or 6 years).

SUBCONJUNCTIVAL HAEMORRHAGES

These and petechiae on the head and neck are common and have no pathological significance.

SUBCUTANEOUS FAT NECROSIS

This produces a firm subcutaneous area at the site of pressure, especially of obstetric forceps. It may be red and tender and aspiration, which is not recommended, may produce yellow material resembling pus. No treatment is required. If the site is unusual and the swelling is not noticed until a few days after birth, it may be confused with a pyogenic abscess.

CHAPTER SIX

Small Infants

DEFINITIONS

Low birth weight infants are 2.5 kg or less. Infants may be small at birth due to a short gestation period or retarded growth rate. When the period of gestation is less than 37 completed weeks the infant is called pre-term. A baby with retarded growth rate is 'light-for-dates' and may be either malnourished or hypoplastic (for example, an infant with a chromosome abnormality). About 30% of babies who have been born early (short gestation period) are also light-for-dates.

The length of gestation, as calculated from the date of the mother's last menstrual period, can be confirmed by a detailed neurological examination of the infant, as the development of the central nervous system is related to the gestational age. Retarded growth is very difficult to assess but valuable signs are the size of the fetus by palpation after the 28th week of pregnancy and a birth weight below the 10th centile for the gestational age (see p.108). Recent ultrasound studies have shown that when intrauterine malnutrition starts early in pregnancy, the head circumference and weight are in the normal proportions, but when the onset is late in pregnancy the head is disproportionately large due to a relatively normal growth of the brain. Retarded growth is often associated with placental insufficiency which may be assessed by falling maternal urinary oestriol levels.

In most respects, the management of the infant is the same whether pre-term or light-for-dates, but the distinction is helpful because certain complications are more likely to occur in one group than the other.

	PRE-TERM	LIGHT-FOR-DATES
Cause	Short gestation	Intrauterine malnutrition (placental insufficiency)
Dangers	Respiratory distress syndrome Hypothermia Infection Intraventricular or subarachnoid haemorrhage	Hypoglycaemia Hypocalcaemia Hypothermia
Length	Crown–heel less than 45 cm	May be more than 45 cm
Head circumference	Less than 33 cm	Often more than 33 cm
Skin	Thin, red	Dry, folds of lax skin
Muscle tone	Poor, frog-like posture	Variable

The head circumference should be compared to the weight using centile charts (see p.108 and 109).

TEMPERATURE

Small infants become hypothermic quickly. Heat loss may be considerable because they have a large surface area in relation to their body weight and there is a deficiency of subcutaneous fat for insulation. Also there is a lack of 'brown fat' which is usually present in the full-term baby and can be metabolised rapidly to produce heat. A high constant environmental temperature is required to avoid hypothermia which is associated with a *raised* metabolic rate and *increased* caloric and oxygen consumption. If it is decided to nurse the infant in an incubator naked to improve observation, excessive heat loss by radiation can be minimised by an additional tunnel of perspex, a heat shield, placed immediately over the infant. For very small infants the temperature of the air near the mattress can be kept more stable by closing one end of the shield with perspex.

Heat loss will be minimised by maintaining a high environmental temperature. The following recommendations for incubator temperatures are based upon the assumption that the room temperature will be 27°C (80°F) which is the highest temperature tolerable to the nursing staff. The infant's rectal temperature should remain about 37°C.

Weight of infant	*Temperature of incubator*
1 kg	35°C (95°F)
2 kg	34°C (93°F)
3 kg	33°C (91°F)

The incubator temperature is reduced by 1°C weekly. When the infant weighs nearly 2 kg (4 lb) he is usually transferred to a cot and later to a cooler room (24°C) before discharge. The recommended incubator temperatures for the smallest infants require the use of specially adjusted incubators. The smallest infants may need a higher incubator temperature than that recommended above.

The risk of hypothermia can be reduced by the use of a gamgee lined hat which can be placed on an infant's head shortly after birth but must be removed when the infant is placed in an incubator.

Hypothermia can be avoided by carrying out resuscitation under a heat lamp or radiant heat canopy, bearing in mind the danger of burns if the lamp is too close. However, if the baby is hypothermic the temperature should be allowed to rise gradually over several hours in a heated environment and no attempt should be made to increase it quickly. Although parents wish to know the infant's weight soon after birth, the risk of hypothermia is reduced if weighing of all infants is postponed for a few hours.

It is possible to nurse small babies under a heat canopy for ease of access but additional water and sodium chloride may be needed.

When an infant is transferred from one hospital to another for special care there is a danger of hypothermia. A swaddler made of aluminium foil has been designed to prevent this and is commercially available, but we have found that wrapping the baby with gamgee wool has been satisfactory. The aluminium swaddler has two dangers. If the infant is cold before being wrapped in it, he may remain cold: if the swaddler containing the infant is placed under a heat canopy, the infant can receive a burn. It is advisable to have a portable incubator kept warm continuously and ready for immediate use.

INFECTION

Gowns and masks are no longer used by the medical staff in many units, nor is it necessary for nurses to wear masks, but a separate plastic apron or gown of waterproof material is used for the nursing of each infant to prevent soiling of the nurse's clothes. Hands should be washed before and after touching each infant, taking care to use elbow taps correctly, but scrubbing with a brush should be avoided. Liberal application of a chlorhexidine cream to the hands after washing, washing the incubators with a chlorhexidine solution and the use of formalin to disinfect incubators are valuable methods of preventing cross infection. If incubators can be left in the open air, less vigorous methods of chemical treatment are necessary. As an additional safeguard the wearing of plastic disposable gloves is advised when changing infants' napkins. Ideally, any infant who develops an infection, should be isolated in a separate nursery and barrier nursed. No member of the staff with an upper respiratory tract or other infection should be allowed to work in the unit. Babies born outside the hospital should be admitted to a separate nursery. Adequate numbers of meticulous nursing staff are probably the most important factor in the prevention of cross infection.

Infection in a small infant may be very insidious and should be suspected if there are any symptoms however slight. If the nursing staff have the slightest anxiety about any infant, even in the absence of abnormal signs, full investigation as for pyrexia is warranted (see p.93).

GESTATIONAL AGE ASSESSMENT

We have given three schemes for assessment. The neurological table (below) is a quick guide but the chart on pp.122–3 or those on pp.117–21 are needed for detailed assessment.

	GESTATION IN COMPLETED WEEKS	
	Present	Absent
Pupil reaction to light	more than 29	less than 31
Glabellar tap	,, ,, 32	,, ,, 34
Traction	,, ,, 33	,, ,, 36
Neck righting	,, ,, 34	,, ,, 37
Head turning to diffuse light	,, ,, 32	,, ,, 36

FEEDING (see p.48)

Pre-term infants have poor sucking and cough reflexes and methods of feeding must prevent aspiration into the lungs. Continuous intragastric drip feeds or frequent feeds of small volume prevent abdominal distension with resultant pressure on the diaphragm and apnoeic attacks. Early feeding prevents hypoglycaemia and reduces the maximum serum bilirubin level. A Dextrostix test is performed on all low birth weight babies 3 hourly for the first 48 h of life. If the test shows a level below 1.4 mmol/l (25 mg/100 ml) the blood glucose level is estimated in the laboratory. Asymptomatic hypoglycaemia is treated initially by feeding with milk and the Dextrostix test is repeated an hour later. If the level is still less than 1.4 mmol/l the blood glucose level is estimated in the laboratory, and a low level (see p.81) is discussed immediately with the paediatrician. From the 2nd week onwards vitamin supplements are added such as ABIDEC 0.6 ml daily; this contains vitamin A 4000 U, vitamin C 50 mg, vitamin D 400 U and small amounts of the vitamin B complex. In addition iron is given as ferrous fumerate.

MATERNAL SEPARATION (see p.55)

CHAPTER SEVEN

Feeding

INTRODUCTION

The principles of feeding newborn babies have been based on observation of large numbers of healthy breast-fed infants. The individual baby may need more or less than the calculated average requirement in order to gain weight at the optimum rate as judged by progress on a growth chart.

A normal full term infant receives 30 ml of milk/kg body weight during the 1st day of feeding by bottle. Feeds are increased by 20 ml/kg each day until a maximum of 150 ml/kg is reached on the 7th day of feeding. If, for any reason, the baby needs more fluid, water can be added to the feeds to increase the volume up to the maximum requirement for day 7.

The birth weight is usually regained between the 7th and 10th day, and thereafter the infant should gain 30 g/day for the next 100 days. Breast milk and the new low solute milks contain the complete vitamin requirements and no supplementary vitamins are needed. Infants who receive other milks should start vitamin supplements at the age of 2 weeks and continue them until 1 year. In areas where nutritional rickets is common, vitamin supplements containing vitamin D are needed for a longer period, at least until the age of 2 years. In these areas vitamin supplements are also given to babies receiving breast milk. Underfeeding causes small amounts of green mucus to be passed frequently and there is poor weight gain. This introduction gives the bare essentials; larger works should be consulted for further details.

BREAST FEEDING

This should be encouraged for the following reasons:

1 Breast feeding is the most certain method of promoting mother–infant attachment (see p.55).

2 The fat and protein of human milk are more easily and completely absorbed than those of cow's milk. Breast milk is a perfectly balanced diet for the growing infant: it is unlikely that a fully breast-fed baby will become obese.

3 Human milk especially the first milk, colostrum, contains antibodies and a special protein (lactoferrin) which may protect the infant against infections. Gastroenteritis is rare among breast fed babies.

4 Exclusive breast feeding for 6 months lessens the risk of hypersensitivity to cow's milk protein.

5 Absence of napkin rashes.

If the mother is encouraged during the antenatal period to expect to be able to breast feed her baby and eventually to obtain enjoyment from it, she is likely to accept early difficulties with patience and understanding. The close contact and intimacy—and often supreme enjoyment of breast feeding—provide the best 'feed-back' from the baby to the mother. The mother's intimate personal relationship with her baby is something which she has to work out for herself. Many feel insecure and inadequate at first and are only too glad to change to bottle feeding whenever the slightest difficulty arises. The attendant should resist the temptation to accede to such requests and instead should use all her sympathy, understanding and skill to encourage the mother to gain confidence in handling her own baby.

A normal infant is put to the breast for a few minutes at each side either immediately or about 6 h after birth. Only a small amount of colostrum is obtained but sucking by the infant stimulates the production of more milk. Some infants are reluctant to take the nipple initially and the mother requires strong reasurrance that this occurs commonly. We suggest that the most satisfactory method of breast feeding is 'on demand'. Babies commonly feed 2 or 3 hourly during the 1st week and these frequent feeds are a powerful stimulus to lactation. This is the main advantage of 'rooming in', where the infant's cot is always by the side of the mother's bed and she is able to pick her baby up and feed him when he cries and the mother should be encouraged to do so. Infants who are initially fed on demand usually settle down to a regular schedule after a few weeks. Some mothers prefer a more rigid schedule and for them we suggest that by the 3rd day the infant should be fed 3 or 4 hourly for 5–10 min on each breast.

After the 4th day, if the infant appears to be hungry after a feed or there is progressive weight loss, test feeding may be considered. Test feeding should be avoided wherever possible as it can create anxiety in some mothers. The infant is weighed without changing the napkin or clothes before and after each feed during a 24 h period. If the amount of feed is deficient, putting the baby to the breast more frequently may stimulate the increased lactation in the early days. Alternatively, the deficit may be made up with bottle feeds (complementary feeding). Fortunately, a well-nourished full term baby can tolerate a degree of underfeeding without harm for several days, especially if given extra water. Complementary feeds are rarely necessary in the first 5 days, and after this they should be used only when absolutely necessary. The feel of the bottle teat is quite different from that of the nipple: when the baby is accustomed to the one it may be difficult to persuade him to take from the other. The introduction of one or two artificial feeds, given by the staff at night, may be enough to break down the barrier to infection provided by breast feeding, and there is evidence that some infants may develop eczema by being exposed to cow's milk protein before immunological competence has been acquired.

There are few contraindications to breast feeding. Some women have a revulsion to the idea and it would be a mistake to try and persuade them, but psychiatric illness in the mother may be aggravated if the baby is taken off the breast. A severely cracked nipple is a temporary contraindication to feeding from the affected breast but feeding can continue from a breast with an early abscess.

No drugs should be taken by a lactating mother unless there are strong clinical indications. Most drugs that are essential for the mother are excreted in the milk in insignificant amounts, so breast feeding should not be stopped unless there is a special reason. Warfarin, senna, barbiturates, phenytoin, digoxin, steroids, sodium valproate and occasional doses of acetyl salicylic acid pass into the milk in insignificant amounts. A mother receiving carbimazole may continue to breast feed provided that the infant's plasma T4 level is monitored. Oestrogens in oral contraceptives may reduce lactation but the progesterone-only pill is an effective contraceptive and has no effect on lactation. Mothers receiving radioactive antithyroid treatment and cytotoxic drugs should not breast feed. Lithium given to the mother may cause hypotonia, hypothermia and episodes of cyanosis in the breast fed infant. Antibiotics are excreted in minute amounts in the milk but there is the theoretical possibility of sensitization of the infant. There may be high levels of drugs in the milk of a mother with renal failure.

BOTTLE FEEDING

In this country the older full cream cow's milk preparations have been replaced by low solute preparations such as SMA, Osterfeed or Premium. These preparations have a sodium and protein content which is similar to that of human milk, and this has reduced the dangers of hypernatraemia, hypocalcaemia and obesity which were associated with the older preparations. The powder should be measured accurately avoiding heaped or packed scoops and the water should be measured before adding it to the powder. (See end of chapter for composition of milks.)

Prepared feeds are being used in many obstetric units, but cannot be obtained for use at home.

If feeds are made up for a 24 h period they should be stored in the refrigerator. Bottles can be sterilised in dilute hypochlorite solution (Milton) but processing in an autoclave is the best method in hospital. The size of the hole in the teat should allow individual drops of milk to follow each other quickly when the bottle is inverted. Feeds are usually given on demand, or 3- to 4-hourly. Few babies can manage without a night feed for the first few months.

TUBE FEEDING

Infants weighing less than 2 kg usually have a poor sucking reflex and tube feeding is necessary to enable the fluid requirements to be given. Infants just above 2 kg may suck well but sometimes it is necessary to give half the feed or the whole of each alternate feed by tube.

Tube feeding may be intermittent or continuous.

Intermittent

Intermittent feeds may need to be given 3 hourly, hourly or even more frequently initially. Suitable PVC tubes are FG3.5 (Argyle) for infants less than 1.75 kg and FG6.0 (Warne) for heavier babies. When the larger tube is used, the milk can be given by gravity rather than syringe and this improves the safety of the method. Water is given 1 h after birth and full strength milk at 2 h. The initial volume is 60 ml/kg body weight per 24 h and this is increased by daily increments of 30 ml/kg to a maximum of 200 ml/kg.

Continuous

Continuous milk drip feeds have many advantages and have gained general acceptance. The risks of hypoglycaemia are minimised, there is less handling of the infant, and less nursing time is required. It is of special value in infants prone to hypoglycaemia, i.e. those below the 10th or above the 90th centile for weight.

The infant is nursed on a firm mattress covered by absorbent material (two thicknesses of paper towelling). It is most important that his position is prone, and it may be advisable to have the head higher than the feet. This not only reduces regurgitation but ensures that if it occurs the milk spills from the mouth and is not aspirated into the lungs.

For infants weighing 1.5–2.5 kg the 4.5 FG PVC tube (Warne) is suitable, but for infants below 1.5 kg the 3.5 FG PVC tube (Argyle) is preferable. The tube is passed through the nose into the stomach; the usual distance is 20 cm but it is best to check the length between the nose, external auditory meatus and lower end of the sternum. The tube adjacent to the nose is marked with strapping. Fluid is aspirated and if it is colourless and acid to litmus, the tube is in the correct position and is taped securely to the cheek with adhesive plaster. If green fluid is obtained, the tube is withdrawn 2 cm and aspiration repeated. Aspiration just before a feed is performed at least three times each 24 h and the tube is changed every 3rd day.

The bottle of milk is attached to a disposable intravenous giving set by using a sterile rubber transfusion bottle bung instead of a teat. The giving set is attached to the feeding tube. The bottle is hung on a dripstand about 1 m above the infant. The bottle is changed every 8 h and the giving set every 24 h. During the first few days, when the volumes are small, a constant infusion pump or a syringe pump can be used, or the milk can be added with a syringe directly to the burette of the giving set. 5% glucose is given at 1 h after birth and continuous milk is started at 2 h.

When milk feeding is started only full strength milk is given, preferably expressed by the mother, otherwise a cow's milk preparation with low protein content, e.g. SMA. For pre-term infants the initial volume is 60 ml/kg body weight per 24 h and this is increased by daily increments of 30 ml/kg to a maximum of 240 ml/kg provided it is well tolerated. If breast milk is being used it is possible to increase the volume to 270 ml/kg per day. These large volumes have not been associated with aspiration pneumonia or hypocalcaemic convulsions in our experience. The rate of weight gain may be faster than the neurological development and tube feeding may still be required for infants when they weigh over 2 kg. However, alternate bottle feeds can be introduced at this stage and complete bottle feeding by the time the infant is of sufficient weight for discharge home.

APPROXIMATE % COMPOSITION OF MILKS

	PROTEIN	FAT	CARBOHYDRATE	MINERALS
Breast milk	1.2	3.8	7.0	0.2
Cow's milk	3.3	3.7	4.8	0.7

Mothers of babies born as early as 28 weeks gestation are capable of breast feeding their babies on discharge, provided their lactation is maintained by expression of milk and later putting the baby to the breast.

INTRAVENOUS FEEDING

Intravenous feeding with glucose, amino acids and lipid has a place in the management of selected infants with necrotising enterocolitis or after extensive resection of the small intestine. There is no convincing evidence that intravenous feeding improves the prognosis for infants of low birth weight and we do not recommend it.

INTRAJEJUNAL FEEDING

Pre-term infants in some units are fed by continuous intrajejunal feeds. The special feeding tube has a weighted end and a radio-opaque line so that the position of the tube can be checked by screening or a straight radiograph. We have found continuous intragastric feeds a simpler technique but equally effective.

CHAPTER EIGHT

Mother–Infant Bonding

There is a fundamental biological need for a close mother–infant attachment to give the infant the degree of security necessary for optimal emotional and physical development.

Some mothers have strong maternal feelings which enable them to achieve a firm bond of affection with their babies without any difficulty, even after an initial period of separation. The strength of their maternal feelings is probably dependent upon the quality of mothering they themselves received in infancy. On the contrary, a mother may be unable to achieve this attachment without early close contact with her baby, and even then it may take a few days before the baby appears to her to be an individual and her own. Failure to form a normal attachment is considered the reason for the higher incidence of 'battered babies' in pre-term infants who were initially separated from their mothers for long periods and in infants of mothers who themselves were deprived of maternal attachment.

HOW DOES ATTACHMENT OCCUR?

1 The infant can follow the mother's eyes immediately after birth and this eye-to-eye contact is an important factor.
2 If a mother is left with her naked infant she touches each part of his body with her finger tips.
3 During the first few days after delivery mothers often appear overprotective to their infants and become what appears to be inappropriately anxious to the minor difficulties such as those of feeding.
4 Physical contact during breast feeding and the presence of the baby next to the mother throughout the entire 24 h also promote attachment.

WHAT INTERFERES?

Separation is sometimes unavoidable, if, for example, the infant has to be transferred to another unit for surgery or the mother is receiving heavy sedation for hypertension. The mother is equally separated from her baby when severely depressed but this may not appear so obvious. In the past many babies were separated from their mothers due to the anxiety of doctors. Some of the reasons would no longer be acceptable such as cot nursing of infants after forceps delivery and the admission of infants with prolonged jaundice to the special care unit, although they needed no special care. The number of nursing staff available on individual maternity wards will determine whether it is safe physically for a baby to remain with his mother, but no infant should be separated from his mother without good reason.

OMINOUS FEATURES

Some aspects of the history may suggest that a particular mother may have difficulty in forming an attachment to her infant and will need special help from the nursing and medical staff. A mother who has requested an abortion which has been rejected, or an unmarried mother who has not decided whether she wishes the infant to be adopted are particularly vulnerable. If a previous infant was stillborn or died in the neonatal period, or the mother is less than 17 years or over 35 years of age and having her first baby, help may be needed. When the baby is born the mother may refuse to handle or feed him and be more concerned with her own minor symptoms than the infant's care. These may be the first symptoms of a severe depression in the mother and psychiatric help may be required.

HOW TO ENCOURAGE ATTACHMENT

The principle is to avoid unnecessary separation. This may involve considerable changes in the organisation of work in the maternity unit. Even if an abnormality such as mongolism is present (see p.38) the infant should be given to his mother in the labour room. The baby is very lively and looks around during the 1st hour after birth, even if the mother has received heavy sedation during labour. He is put to the breast if the mother intends to breast feed. The infant should remain with the mother throughout the 24 h and only be taken out at night if the other mothers in the room are continually disturbed by him. Breast feeding should be actively encouraged, appreciating that it may take time and perseverance by both mothers and nursing staff (see p.50). Mothers of pre-term infants should be encouraged to express their milk and thus feel that they are actively contributing to the infant's welfare.

In special care units the atmosphere should make mothers feel that they are welcome at any time and they should be encouraged to look at, touch, change, feed and later breast feed their infants. If the mother is about to visit a very sick infant, the reasons for the use of special apparatus should be explained beforehand. A mother can usually visit her infant in the special care unit the day after a Caesarian section by being wheeled in a chair by her husband. If the mother fails to visit the infant for long periods after she has been discharged, an enquiry should be made whether any remediable reason such as lack of transport is responsible. Weekly meetings of the whole unit and occasional case conferences may enable some of these problems to be resolved at an early stage. Before the infant is discharged from the unit the mother should remain with her infant in a room on the unit for at least 24 h but longer if possible. This gives her an opportunity to gain confidence in her ability to cope with her baby who recently appeared to the mother to be so fragile and needing expert nursing care to survive.

CHAPTER NINE

Vomiting

DEFINITION

The expulsion of gastric contents through the mouth.

CLINICAL FEATURES

The character of the material vomited and the time of the vomit in relation to the feed may help to limit the number of possible diagnoses. Often the vomit contains only milk, but a careful history and examination enables a diagnosis to be made with the minimum of special investigations.

TYPES OF VOMIT

Frothy mucoid

Oesophageal atresia with tracheo-oesophageal fistula may present with vomiting, coughing and cyanosis when the infant begins the first feed. Vomiting of *frothy* mucoid material may be the only definite observation reported, but the condition should be suspected in any baby who has *any* symptoms during the first feed. As the fluid expelled is not gastric contents, vomiting is not an accurate description but this is the term often used. Duodenal atresia or anorectal malformation may also be present in infants with oesophageal atresia.

Bile stained

The vomitus of intestinal obstruction is usually green due to bile staining but occasionally consists only of milk. The cause may be atresia, stenosis or volvulus of the small gut necrotising enterocolitis or congenital intestinal aganglionosis (Hirschsprung's disease) of the large gut. Abdominal distension is often present and there may be visible peristalsis. Plain radiographs of the abdomen in the erect, supine and lateral positions should be taken immediately. They often show fluid levels, dilated loops of gut proximal to the obstruction and absence of gas shadows distally. Duodenal atresia has the characteristic 'double bubble appearance' radiologically. If the infant is too ill to be taken out of the incubator, the erect radiograph can be replaced by a film taken with the infant lying on his back or side and the X-ray tube placed at the side of the incubator. Ideally every infant who vomits bile should be seen by a surgeon within 1 h.

Blood

1 Haemorrhagic disease of the newborn begins between the 2nd and 4th days of life. The first symptoms may be haematemesis or melaena and the bleeding may be rapid and profuse. Pallor and increase in the heart rate at rest indicate significant blood loss. Treatment consists of giving an immediate dose of vitamin K_1 (1 mg) intramuscularly and transfusing blood if bleeding has been severe. If the signs suggest that haemorrhage has been profuse it may be necessary to give group O rhesus negative blood without cross-matching. This blood should be as fresh as possible. The fresh blood provides the deficient clotting factors as well as correcting the fall in blood volume and the anaemia. An initial infusion of 10 ml/kg body weight can be repeated once if further bleeding occurs. Reliable statistical surveys have shown that the incidence of haemorrhagic disease of the newborn can be drastically reduced by giving every newborn infant, independent of weight, 1 mg of vitamin K_1 intramuscularly once.

2 Maternal blood may be swallowed before delivery following premature separation of the placenta during delivery, or after delivery as a result of bleeding from a cracked nipple. Maternal haemoglobin in the vomit can be recognised in the laboratory by the ability of alkali to denature it.

3 Trauma by a feeding tube may produce a few specks of blood in the vomit.

4 Volvulus of small gut may be associated with the vomiting of dark blood.

5 Hiatus hernia (see p.62).

Milk

1 Infection. (a) Gastroenteritis. Newborn infants with gastroenteritis rarely vomit but in such cases vomiting may precede diarrhoea for as long as 48 h (see p.63); (b) urinary infection (see p.102); (c) septicaemia (see p.101); (d) meningitis (see p.101).

2 Feeding problems. A ravenous infant may swallow excessive air at the beginning of a feed, and if the infant is not properly 'winded', milk may be regurgitated later with air. Larger feeds or a larger hole in the teat are needed. In light-for-dates infants receiving large volumes of full strength feed to prevent hypoglycaemia, thick curds may obstruct the pylorus of the small gut ('the milk plug syndrome'), causing abdominal distension and vomiting. It will be necessary to carry out gastric lavage using syringefuls of 0.9% sodium chloride solution with an FG9 tube and give feeds of clear fluid followed by gradually increasing strengths of milk. It is important to seek surgical advice without delay to exclude, for example, intestinal obstruction due to a congenital abnormality (see p.59).

3 Necrotising enterocolitis. The early symptoms are lethargy and refusal of feeds followed by vomiting and abdominal distension. In at least 25% of the infants blood is passed *per rectum*. There has been an increased incidence of this condition in some units. The predisposing factors are prematurity, perinatal hypoxia, hypotension, umbilical vessel catheterisation and prolonged rupture of the membranes. Embolism or thrombosis of mesenteric vessels are followed by ischaemic changes which vary from mucosal ulceration to complete necrosis of the gut wall. Bacteria invade the necrotic tissue and healing is followed by scarring and sometimes a stricture. Any part of the gut may be affected but the ileum and colon are most commonly involved. An abdominal mass or oedema of the abdominal wall suggests that perforation of the gut has occurred. An erect radiograph of the abdomen may show air under the diaphragm, confirming perforation, or the characteristic sign of intramural gas. After taking blood for culture, intravenous fluids are started and gastric aspiration is performed at regular intervals. Penicillin is given intravenously and gentamicin intramuscularly. A surgeon should be consulted at an early stage. Laparotomy may be indicated if there is evidence of perforation. No oral fluids are given for at least a week and intravenous feeding may be indicated (see p.114). Despite optimal treatment, necrotising entercolitis has a 50% mortality rate.

4 Raised intracranial pressure due to intracranial haemorrhage.

5 Drugs, especially digoxin (see p.132).

6 Duodenal obstruction presents with vomiting of milk without bile if the lesion is proximal to the entrance of the common bile duct into the duodenum.

RARE CAUSES OF NEONATAL VOMITING

1 Inguinal hernia is more liable to incarcerate in the newborn period than later in life. Incarceration should be suspected if the hernia is tender or is not reduced easily, and immediate surgery is required.

The risk of obstruction is always present and early surgical treatment is advised in every baby with an inguinal hernia. The baby must remain in the ward until the operation is performed.

2 The adrenogenital syndrome (salt-losing type) commonly presents with vomiting as the only symptom in the male; the diagnosis is rendered easier in the female by the virilisation of the external genitalia and a chromatin positive buccal smear. Symptoms usually begin about the 10th day and may be fatal within a few hours if extra salt and salt-retaining adrenocortical steroids are not given. Intravenous fluids are required. The diagnosis is confirmed by a high plasma potassium, low plasma sodium and raised urinary ketosteroids. However, the serum electrolytes are normal at birth and marked changes may occur suddenly.

3 Pyloric stenosis is not a rare abnormality but pre-term babies are liable to remain in hospital until the 3rd week of life when the disease usually presents. Any baby aged between 10 days and 2 months who vomits may have pyloric stenosis. Palpation of a pyloric tumour during a test feed is pathognomonic and preliminary aspiration and measurement of gastric contents is helpful.

4 Hiatus hernia may present at any age but there is frequently a history of vomiting from birth and the vomit is occasionally blood-stained. It is necessary to exclude all the causes of vomiting noted above before this diagnosis is considered. The diagnosis should be confirmed by a barium swallow examination. It is a common practice to keep the infant sitting upright by special techniques both day and night. If the infant is under the age of 3 months this has many disadvantages such as the production of deformities of the skull and pelvis. At this age it is preferable to nurse the infant prone on a firm surface at an angle of 30–45° with the head higher than the trunk.

Diarrhoea

DEFINITION

The too frequent passage of too loose stools.

CLINICAL FEATURES

A stool should be observed personally. A rectal examination or the passage of a rectal thermometer is often followed by a fresh stool which can be examined. When diarrhoea is severe, the stools may be mistaken for urine. When this is a possibility, a urine bag should be placed in position and the infant nursed on a sheet of polythene.

The normal stools of a breast-fed infant are never formed, may be passed frequently, contain mucus, and may be green in colour. When lactation becomes established between the 3rd and 5th days, intestinal hurry is common with resulting frequent stools. Later they tend to become less frequent and more pasty in consistency and by the age of 3 weeks may be passed once every 2 or 3 days.

CAUSES

Breast-fed infants

1 Laxatives, e.g. cascara taken by the mother. Senna does not have this effect as it is not transferred to the milk.
2 Starvation stools. These consist of frequent *small* amounts of dark green mucoid material.

Gastroenteritis is very rare in wholly breast-fed infants.

Bottle-fed infants

1 Gastroenteritis. The chief dangers are cross infection and dehydration. Stool specimens are cultured but can be expected to produce a bacterial pathogen in less than 15% of patients with gastroenteritis. The most common bacterial pathogen is pathogenic *E.coli*. The majority of these babies have a virus of the rotavirus group which can be detected by electron microscopy. Isolation and barrier nursing are essential and if dehydration is severe, as shown by a weight loss of 10% or more or there is severe diarrhoea, intravenous fluids are given.

We use scalp vein infusions with the butterfly 25 gauge short needle but a 23 gauge is needed for blood. A special paediatric intravenous giving set must be used for accurate measurement of the volume administered. An infusion pump, for example IVAC or syringe pump, is essential in ensuring a constant rate of flow. The site of the needle must be checked frequently as the pump will continue delivering fluid even if the needle is outside the vein. Sodium chloride (0.45%) with 2.5% glucose solution is given at a fast rate until dilute urine has been passed and then 0.18% sodium chloride and glucose solution with potassium supplements at a slower rate (see p.113).

If the plasma sodium level is above 155 mmol/l (155 m equiv/l) (severe hypernatraemia) there is a danger of convulsions during rehydration and further advice should be sought at an early stage. Marked metabolic acidosis with a plasma bicarbonate level less than 12 mmol/l (12 m equiv/l) should be partially corrected (see p.113).

In less severe cases, or after 24 h of intravenous therapy in severely dehydrated infants, oral 0.18% sodium chloride with 4% glucose and 1.5 g potassium chloride per litre is given for 24 h and milk feeds in gradually increasing strengths introduced over the subsequent 5 days. If two or more infants have diarrhoea at the same time, even if the stool cultures show no pathogens, cross infection is presumed. Stools from all the infants in the ward are sent for culture and electron microscopy. Antibiotics are mainly useful in reducing cross infection and should not be given without further advice. Depending on the severity of the symptoms and the number of infants involved, it may be necessary to stop admissions to the ward.

A small number of infants have a recurrence of diarrhoea

after the reintroduction of milk. If the stool fluid contains over 0.5% of reducing substances when tested with *Clinitest*, a specimen should be sent to the laboratory for sugar chromatography. Secondary lactose intolerance may be the cause for the diarrhoea and the symptoms may be alleviated by giving a lactose-free milk, for example Galactomin 17, for a few weeks. Vitamin supplements are needed and can be given as Ketovite liquid together with Ketovite tablets which are lactose- and sucrose-free.

The testing of the stool with *Clinitest* should be performed in a disposable tube, for example a universal container, to avoid contamination of the nurse's hands with potentially infected material.

Small amounts of lactulose produced during sterilisation of prepared fluid feed may produce symptoms similar to those of lactose intolerance. In these patients it may be necessary to use dried powdered milk rather than prepared feeds.

Either breast- or bottle-fed

1 Drugs: penicillins and iron.
2 Urinary infection (see p.102).
3 Hirschsprung's disease usually presents as a 'late starter'. The first passage of meconium is delayed until after 24 h following birth but diarrhoea is rarely the first symptom.

CHAPTER ELEVEN

Breathing Difficulties

CAUSES

Primary or secondary pulmonary conditions or disorders of the central nervous system.

CLINICAL FEATURES

Pulmonary lesions are associated with a rapid respiratory rate sometimes with an expiratory grunt, intercostal recession and sternal retraction. Disorders of the central nervous system cause apnoea, slow gasping respirations or periodic breathing.

PULMONARY CAUSES

Respiratory distress syndrome (RDS)

Pre-term babies are particularly susceptible, but it also occurs in the obese infants of mothers with diabetes mellitus or prediabetes.

Anoxia before or after birth is a predisposing factor and may be the reason for the increased incidence following Caesarian section in some series.

The cause is a deficiency of pulmonary surfactant, a substance normally present on the alveolar walls which has the remarkable property of lowering the surface tension in the alveoli in such a way that, whatever their size, the same pressure is required to inflate them all. This enables easy and uniform inflation of all alveoli. Surfactant also prevents the alveolar walls from collapsing during expiration. Without surfactant, the surface tension is very great in the smaller alveoli causing them to collapse, whereas larger alveoli continue to expand easily; thus there is uneven expansion with increasingly widespread alveolar collapse. Surfactant production in the fetal lung is poor before the 34th week of gestation and the level in the fetal lung correlates well with the L/S ratio in the amniotic fluid (see p.2).

The incidence of respiratory distress syndrome increases with decreasing gestation so that at 27–31 weeks 35–50% of all infants are affected. About three out of every 1000 infants born alive die from respiratory distress syndrome. Postmortem examination frequently shows on microscopy the presence of amorphous material lining the terminal bronchioles and alveoli which is called hyaline membrane. In addition there are multiple areas of alveolar collapse.

An expiratory grunt, a respiratory rate over 60/min and recession of the chest wall begin within 3 h of birth. Central cyanosis in air and oedema of the limbs may appear later. Usually auscultation of the lungs reveals only reduced breath sounds, but crepitations may be present. In the majority of infants in the early stages of the disease the chest X-ray shows normal lung fields but later a fine reticular pattern or generalised loss of translucency ('the ground glass appearance') may be present. The contrast between the air in the bronchi and the opaque lung fields produces an air bronchogram. The greatest value of the chest X-ray is in excluding other conditions which will be mentioned later.

MANAGEMENT

Nursing

The infant should be handled as little as possible. Abrupt deterioration in the clinical state may result from moving the infant during frequent recording of rectal temperature or changing of sheets. The infant is best nursed in the prone position with the head inclined upwards. This does not interfere with respiratory movements and the presence of umbilical catheters is not usually a contraindication but some authorities prefer nursing the infant on the side or back.

Oxygen

Oxygen measurement. During oxygen therapy the arterial oxygen tension (PaO_2) should not fall below 6.7 kPa (50 mm Hg) with the risk of anoxic brain damage or rise above 12.0 kPa (90 mm Hg) with the possibility of retrolental fibroplasia and subsequent blindness. Some infants may require high concentrations of inhaled oxygen to prevent hypoxia but this can only be given safely if facilities for frequent PaO_2 estimations are available continuously. Arterial blood oxygen tension can be measured in samples of blood taken at regular intervals from an umbilical artery catheter. The indications for the insertion of an arterial umbilical catheter vary between units but we include the infant with deteriorating signs or a PaO_2 less than 6.7 kPa (50 mm Hg) when the oxygen concentration in the head-box is 40% or more.This initial blood oxygen concentration can be estimated by a sample obtained by radial artery puncture or by using a transcutaneous oxygen electrode (see below). If a limb, or part of a limb becomes blue during the insertion of an umbilical catheter, the catheter should be withdrawn slightly. Other dangers include thrombosis, embolism and septicaemia. If the catheter is used for a continuous infusion of fluids, heparin should be added to the fluid at a concentration of 1 i.u./ml. Where the catheter is used solely for sampling, the heparin concentration should be 10 i.u./ml in sodium chloride solution. Some units have found that spraying the catheter insertion site once with a mixture of antibiotics which are not absorbed has reduced the incidence of infection at the umbilicus. The 5 FG catheter has a capacity of 0.2 ml and the volume of all blood samples should be measured as a blood transfusion is needed when 5–10 ml of blood, depending on the infant's weight, has been removed.

Another approach is the use of an oxygen-sensitive electrode which is incorporated into the tip of the umbilical artery catheter. This has the advantage that the oxygen levels are measured continuously but the electrode must be calibrated at regular intervals by estimating the oxygen tension in samples of blood aspirated through the lumen of the catheter.

The transcutaneous oxygen electrode has recently been introduced in several units. The heated electrode increases the blood flow to the skin where the oxygen tension is measured. The electrode must be moved every 4 h to avoid burns but the method has the advantages that it is not invasive and the electrode is calibrated with a gas mixture.

Oxygen Treatment. An outline of the indications for the

various methods of treatment is shown in Fig.4. A perspex Gairdner head-box with venturi can be used to provide constant oxygen concentrations above that in air. The venturi attachment draws warm air from the incubator into the headbox with the cold oxygen preventing the infant from being cooled. If the incubator is humidified the oxygen is humidified by mixing with the air drawn by the venturi, otherwise a humidifier should be inserted in the oxygen supply. The oxygen sensor is placed near the infant's mouth and the oxygen concentration should be measured at least once an hour; calculations from oxygen flow rates are unreliable.

Fluids

A full strength milk mixture may be given by continuous gastric drip at the rate of 60 ml/kg of body weight in each 24 h. Alternatively small volumes of feed can be given intermittently at frequent intervals (see p.52). The volume is increased by increments of 30 ml/kg/24 h until a maximum of 180 ml/kg in each 24 h is given.

During intermittent positive pressure ventilation, with an endotracheal tube in place, it is safe to continue intragastric feeds. When the infant is being weaned from the ventilator or in a severely dyspnoeic infant most units prefer to stop intragastric feeds and give intravenous fluids only. The

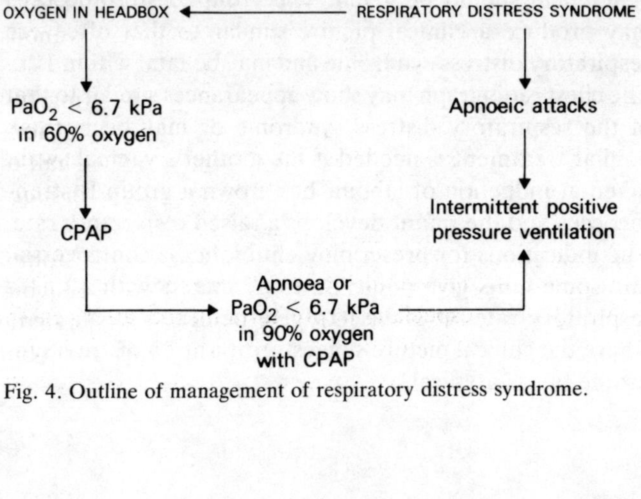

Fig. 4. Outline of management of respiratory distress syndrome.

volumes of the intravenous fluid are similar to the oral feed but with a maximum of 140 ml/kg in 24 h. A suitable solution is 4% glucose and 0.18% sodium chloride with supplementary potassium chloride at a concentration of 20 mmol/l. In the past, many of these infants received plain glucose solutions but this can cause severe hyponatraemia especially in very small pre-term infants.

Infants with an umbilical artery catheter inserted for oxygen measurements can receive fluids through the catheter. The fluid must contain heparin at a concentration of 1 i.u./ml. It is safer to give antibiotics or other substances by another route.

If the PaO_2 is maintained at adequate levels, the pH of the blood is usually maintained at normal levels. In severely ill infants acidosis may occur and it has been a common practice to give sodium bicarbonate solution in amounts which varied with the pH of the blood. Improvements in the management of the respiratory distress syndrome have made this treatment obsolete. The use of sodium bicarbonate solution may be a factor in the aetiology of intraventricular haemorrhage.

Antibiotics

If there is any evidence of infected liquor, prolonged rupture of the membranes, or rapidly progressive disease, intravenous penicillin in high dosage and intramuscular gentamicin should be given. The group B streptococcus may produce a clinical picture similar to that of severe respiratory distress syndrome and may be fatal within 12h. The chest radiograph may show appearances similar to that of the respiratory distress syndrome or may be normal. Similar treatment is needed if the mother's vaginal swab, taken at induction of labour, has grown a group B streptococcus and the infant develops a raised respiratory rate. The indications for prescribing antibiotics is controversial and some units give penicillin to all infants with a raised respiratory rate. It is wise to give penicillin in all cases where the clinical picture suggests respiratory distress syndrome but is atypical.

Continuous Positive Airways Pressure (CPAP)

Several different techniques are being used and the principle is that a low positive pressure is maintained in the alveoli during expiration thus preventing their collapse. The pressure required, if measured at the mouth, is usually 0.3–0.8 kPa (3–8 cm water). The arterial oxygen tension rises with this treatment and lower inhaled oxygen concentrations are needed. The positive pressure can be delivered to the infant by a face mask (held in place by Netelast), or by nasal prongs or an endotracheal tube. We have found the Argyle nasal cannula satisfactory and easy to use. The positive pressure can be generated by a special pump or by a ventilator. Another technique, the Gregory box, provides a positive pressure inside a perspex headbox by a pump supplying a high flow of air or oxygen which is warmed and humidified.

Although it is generally agreed that CPAP should be used before apnoeic attacks occur, the exact indications are controversial. We start CPAP if the PaO_2 is less than 6.7 kPa (50 mmHg) when the infant is in an oxygen concentration of 60%. Arterial oxygen concentration *must* be estimated every 4–6 h in every infant treated with CPAP. Some units have reported very low mortality rates for respiratory distress syndrome when CPAP has been started at an early stage in the disease. Another term for CPAP is constant distending pressure (CDP) or continuous inflating pressure (CIP).Some units have found that CPAP is associated with an increased incidence of pneumothorax which may be as high as 20%. The most common cause of pneumothorax is failure to use only the minimum pressure required.

Intermittent Positive Pressure Ventilation (IPPV)

Repeated apnoeic attacks are an indication that this form of treatment is needed. The other main indications are a PaO_2 less than 6.7 kPa (50 mmHg) or a $PaCO_2$ more than 10 kPa (75 mmHg) when the infant is receiving CPAP and 90% oxygen. Infection and displacement of the endotracheal tube are constant hazards. Fibrosis of the lung has followed later in a small number of infants and was probably due to the high pressures used rather than the high concentrations of oxygen. In view of the dangers of the treatment it should only be undertaken in units where there are adequate nursing and medical staff and enough patients for an effective service to be provided. Larger works should be consulted for details but some practical points follow.

PROBLEM	PROBABLE CAUSE	ACTION
PaO_2 low		
High $PaCO_2$	(a) Ventilator problem	Check O_2 supply and connections
	(b) Infant problem	Consider blocked or displaced endotracheal tube or pneumothorax
Normal $PaCO_2$	Intrapulmonary shunting	Increase end expiratory pressure or increase inspired O_2
$PaCO_2$ low	Excessive ventilation	Decrease rate Rarely increase dead space
$PaCO_2$ high	Underventilation	Depends on ventilator (a) increase peak inflation pressure or (b) increase tidal volume or (c) adjust rate

1 The ventilator should be set initially to give a rate of 30 cycles/min with an inspiratory to expiratory ratio of 1.5:1. The inflating pressure should be 25 cm water (20 mmHg) with a peak end expiratory pressure of 4 cm water (3 mmHg).

2 Both sides of the chest should move equally and breath sounds should be equal on each side.

3 The end of the endotracheal tube should be just above the carina (T5) and must be checked by radiograph.

4 Oro-endotracheal tubes can be held in place using a disposable tracheostomy tube as a 'collar'.
5 Naso-endotracheal tubes may be preferred and suitable connections are commercially available.

Management of Patent Ductus Arteriosus
It has been claimed that the increasing number of very small infants who have survived after treatment with intermittent positive pressure ventilation has been associated with an increased incidence of infants with heart failure due to patent ductus arteriosus. These infants have a raised respiratory rate, enlarged liver and a long, loud systolic murmur. This may continue into diastole and is heard below the left clavicle and is conducted down the left edge of the sternum and to the back. Often the peripheral pulses will be easily palpable.

A significant left to right shunt through the patent ductus arteriosus is conformed if echocardiography shows that the ratio of the left atrial diameter to aorta is greater than 1.5 to 1.0. Digoxin and frusemide are given initially but if severe symptoms persist further measures are considered. It has been suggested that if the infant is less than 2 weeks of age indomethacin can be given orally or rectally in a dosage of 0.1–0.3 mg/kg body weight. One dose is often effective but it may be necessary to repeat the dose after each 24 h to a maximum of three doses. If indomethacin is not effective or the infant is more than 2 weeks of age surgical ligation of the patent ductus arteriosus should be considered.

In our experience heart failure due to patent ductus arteriosus is rare after treatment with intermittent positive pressure ventilation. These patients have usually recovered with no specific treatment or after receiving digoxin and a diuretic. We suspect that a factor in the production of heart failure in these infants may be the giving of more than 140 ml/kg of intravenous fluid in 24 h.

Transient tachypnoea of the newborn (Avery's syndrome)
Raised respiratory rate and grunting from birth or within 3 h is sometimes found in full term infants and resolves

within 48 h. The chest radiograph often shows a streaky appearance in the lung fields but may be normal. Oxygen may be needed. This syndrome may be due to failure of normal reabsorption of lung fluid at birth or a mild form of respiratory distress syndrome.

Pneumothorax

Although this can follow intermittent positive pressure ventilation during the course of resuscitation of an asphyxiated baby, it may occur as the result of the vigorous spontaneous respiratory efforts of such an infant. It can also occur during CPAP or intermittent positive pressure ventilation. A common cause is the displacement of the endotracheal tube into the right main bronchus. *Pneumothorax should be suspected in any infant who deteriorates rapidly for no obvious reason.* It results from overinflation and rupture of alveoli, usually from the effort to overcome an airways obstruction, but there may be an underlying abnormality such as hypoplasia of the lungs. Asymptomatic pneumothorax requires no therapy. When symptoms are present the onset of dyspnoea may be gradual or sudden and the chest may be asymmetrical with bulging of the intercostal spaces on the affected side. There may be hyper-resonance, reduced breath sounds on the affected side and displacement of the heart and mediastinum to the opposite side. Often there are no specific signs but the diagnosis can be made by transilluminating each side of the chest with a powerful fibre-optic light source. Chest X-ray confirms the diagnosis, the absence of normal lung markings being the most important sign.

If the symptoms are severe a disposable cannula is inserted into the pleural space at the fourth intercostal space in the anterior axillary line and is connected to an underwater seal. We use a disposable trocar and cannula (FG 12) and any sterile container with sterile water can be used as an underwater seal in an emergency. We have found that a Heimlich disposable valve is more convenient than an underwater seal. These valves are made in only one size and are suitable for both adults and newborn infants.

It should be remembered that there may be a pneumothorax on each side. Mediastinal emphysema can occur with or without pneumothorax. An unusual elevation of the thymus on the PA chest X-ray is suggestive but the diagnosis is best confirmed by a left lateral film.

Diaphragmatic hernia

In addition to a raised respiratory rate there may be vomiting and a flat appearance of the abdomen. There may be a normal or impaired percussion note and normal or decreased breath sounds whilst bowel sounds may be audible over the chest wall. Since diaphragmatic hernia is most commonly left-sided, it should be suspected in apparent dextrocardia. The chest X-ray may show loops of small gut or solid organs in the thorax. It may take 12 h from birth for air to reach the colon and produce the characteristic appearance. As soon as the diagnosis is made, a wide bore tube, e.g. FG 9, is passed into the stomach and the gastric contents and air are aspirated. This tube is left in place without a spigot and is aspirated at regular intervals. If there is severe dyspnoea after gastric aspiration, intubation is performed preferably by an anaesthetist as there is an increased risk of pneumothorax due to a hypoplastic lung. Intubation should be performed before an ambulance journey as rapid deterioration may occur and intubation is extremely difficult in a moving vehicle.

Congenital lobar emphysema

This may present at any time but is seen most commonly in the neonatal period. There is usually a very high respiratory rate and often central cyanosis. The chest X-ray shows overdistension of one lobe with herniation of the lung across the midline and depression of the diaphragm. The heart and the entire mediastinum are pushed across to the opposite side and there is compression collapse of the unaffected lung.

Lobar emphysema may result from an abnormality of the cartilaginous rings surrounding one of the major bronchi to a lobe. The unsupported bronchial walls collapse and cause a 'check valve' obstruction: with powerful inspiratory efforts air is forced past the obstruction but cannot be expelled, and the lobe becomes greatly overexpanded.

If the X-ray film of the affected lobe clearly shows the presence of lung markings a tension pneumothorax is excluded, but interpretation of the film is often difficult. Emergency thoracotomy and lobectomy are required in most cases where there is severe dyspnoea but mild cases improve spontaneously. There is an association of emphysema of the left upper lobe with some cases of patent ductus arteriosus.

Congenital heart disease

Dyspnoea during feeding, reluctance to feed and a rapid respiratory rate with recession may indicate heart failure. Excessive weight gain and enlargement of the liver are early confirmatory signs. (The edge of the liver is normally about 2 cm below the costal margin in the right midclavicular line.) There may be no murmurs with some lesions; for example, transposition of the great arteries or anomalous pulmonary venous drainage. The diagnosis of congenital heart disease should be strongly suspected in an infant with a cardiac murmur or when central cyanosis is not relieved immediately by 100% oxygen. Oedema of the face and feet is common in normal premature infants and is a late sign of heart failure. Transient heart failure may occur in infants with no cardiac anomalies. It is due to a variety of factors such as difficulty in adapting from the fetal to the neonatal circulation with persistence of fetal pulmonary hypertension, excessive placental transfusion or glycogen depletion of cardiac muscle in light-for-dates babies (see p.43).

Atelectasis

This is failure of the lungs to expand after birth. It occurs especially in pre-term infants after cerebral birth trauma. Difficult resuscitation after birth is immediately followed by a raised respiratory rate, recession and reduced breath sounds on auscultation. The symptoms may persist for as long as 24 h, and oxygen therapy may be indicated. Collapse of part of a lung which has been expanded previously is sometimes called secondary atelectasis but this is a misuse of the word and is best avoided.

Pneumonia

ANTENATAL

Rupture of the membranes for longer than 24 h may be followed by genital tract infection in the mother. Inhalation of infected liquor by the infant may cause pneumonia before birth. Antibiotics such as penicillin which are given to the mother cross the placenta and may begin to combat pulmonary infection before delivery. If the membranes were ruptured over 24h before delivery or the liquor is offensive, the following specimens should be obtained from the newborn infant at birth for culture: gastric aspirate, ear swab, throat swab and umbilical cord swab. If a mother has had ruptured membranes for over 24h before delivery, antibiotics should be considered for the baby in order to prevent or treat pneumonia due to the inhalation of infected liquor.

The group B streptococcus can cause a rapidly progressive septicaemia and pneumonia shortly after birth or a more insidious septicaemia and meningitis towards the end of the 1st week. The presenting features are a raised respiratory rate and the chest radiograph may show extensive areas of consolidation in both lungs or may appear normal. The organism may have been cultured from a vaginal swab before delivery but the mother often has no symptoms. As soon as the chest X-ray and blood culture have been taken, intravenous penicillin and intramuscular gentamicin should be started.

ASPIRATION OF MECONIUM

Infants who become anoxic before delivery may start respiratory movements before there has been an opportunity to clear the mouth and pharynx. The resultant aspiration of meconium may cause bronchial obstruction with secondary collapse and subsequent infection of the distal segments of the lung. In some units the high mortality has been reduced by bronchial lavage at initial resuscitation but this needs considerable skill. Clinically and radiologically it may be difficult to distinguish meconium aspiration from atelectasis. Oxygen and antibiotics are often needed and mechanical ventilation may be required for a few days but complete recovery may take a further 2 weeks.

ASPIRATION OF MILK

Pre-term infants have a poor cough reflex and material such as regurgitated milk in the pharynx is easily aspirated into the lungs, and may cause pneumonia. Signs may be minimal and are often limited to a small increase in the respiratory rate, but a chest X-ray may show extensive changes. Aspiration may be prevented by nursing infants prone so that regurgitated milk spills out of the mouth instead of remaining in the pharynx. The head should be tilted upwards to allow gravity to assist in keeping the gastric contents in the stomach. Penicillin and gentamicin are given. It is often impossible to determine whether bronchopneumonia is primary or secondary to aspiration of milk or meconium, but the treatment is the same. Rarely a tracheo-oesophageal fistula, especially when it occurs without oesophageal atresia, produces no gross symptoms during the first feed and the infant presents with pneumonia due to milk passing through the fistula. Usually, however, babies with this anomaly have choking and coughing spasms at the commencement of each feed.

Severe anaemia

The acute onset of severe anaemia causes a raised respiratory rate. Thus, a strikingly pale dyspnoeic infant at birth demands a haemoglobin estimation and if this is low, immediate blood transfusion is required to prevent death. Oxygen should be given even in the absence of cyanosis.

Choanal atresia or stenosis

Congenital obstruction to air passing through the nose causes the newborn infant considerable difficulty as he depends upon a clear nasal airway. Choanal atresia is a posterior nasal obstruction. There is submandibular recession and lack of movement of a wisp of cotton wool held at the nostril on each side. A rubber or plastic oropharyngeal airway taped to the cheek produces immediate improvement and an ENT surgeon should be consulted, although immediate operation is not indicated.

CENTRAL NERVOUS SYSTEM

Drugs

Morphine or pethidine given to the mother before delivery may cause apnoea in the newborn. Intubation and positive pressure ventilation are the first measures to be taken but it may be necessary to give a chemical antagonist to morphine and to pethidine (see p.18).

Cerebral birth trauma

This may inhibit the onset of spontaneous respiratory movements after birth so that it is necessary to intubate the baby and initiate positive pressure ventilation. Often, however, there are no symptoms until 48 h after delivery when an apnoeic attack occurs, i.e. cessation of respiratory movements lasting over 15 s, perhaps leading on to cyanosis and convulsions. When respiratory movements recommence they are often slow and gasping or have a pattern of increasing and decreasing depth (periodic breathing). These symptoms are due to raised intracranial pressure and are non-specific. (Premature infants without gross pathology often have irregular respiratory movements or periodic breathing.) Similar clinical features occur in hypoxaemia or hypoglycaemia and a Dextrostix test and, if necessary, a blood glucose estimation should be performed. Lumbar puncture will be required to exclude meningitis. When the anterior fontanelle tension is raised and lumbar puncture has excluded meningitis, the possibility of subdural or intraventricular haemorrhage should be considered. A CAT brain scan (computerised axial tomography) may be helpful to determine the presence and site of the haemorrhage.

Apnoea of prematurity

This occurs in infants of very short gestational age. It often begins 24 h after birth and the initial management involves constant observation and flicking the feet whenever an apnoeic attack occurs. It may be necessary to observe the baby for several days and this may be facilitated by the use of an apnoea warning device consisting of a special mattress or a capsule attached to the abdominal wall. If a heart rate meter (or oscilloscope) is available significant apnoeic attacks can be detected reliably because they cause a fall in heart rate.

Recurrent apnoeic attacks may be difficult to manage and may be followed by cerebral palsy at a later date if the episodes are prolonged. Different centres have found the following methods helpful:

1 Raising the inhaled oxygen concentration to 30%. There is a constant danger of retrolental fibroplasia if the concentration rises above 40%. The sensor of an oxygen analyser must remain next to the infant's mouth and the oxygen concentration should be measured once every hour. The use of a transcutaneous oxygen electrode (see p.68) increases the safety of this method of treatment.

2 Aminophylline. The blood levels must be estimated to obtain optimum effects. If aminophylline is given intravenously, one dose of 5 mg/kg body weight lasts for 24 h. The drug should be given slowly over half an hour preferably with a syringe pump. The oral dose is 8 mg/kg body weight per 24 h given in four divided doses 6-hourly, but it may cause vomiting. The optimal blood level is 8–12 μg/ml.

3 CPAP using low pressures (see p.71).

4 Intermittent positive pressure ventilation using low pressures.

When called to see a premature baby who is cyanosed and convulsing, it is worth remembering that these symptoms may have resulted from a prolonged apnoeic attack.

Hypoxaemia

This may cause apnoeic attacks in the acute phase. Aspirated pharyngeal material blocking a main bronchus is a common cause and pharyngeal suction, physiotherapy and antibiotics are required. Hypoxaemia occurs in severe respiratory distress syndrome.

CHAPTER TWELVE

Convulsions

DEFINITION

Repetitive jerky movements which may be accompanied by loss of consciousness, apnoea or rigidity.

AETIOLOGY

1 Hypoglycaemia in the newborn which is represented by a true plasma glucose level (glucose oxidase method) below 1.1 mmol/l (20 mg/100ml). It occurs particularly during the first 72 h of life in babies who are light-for-dates, but may develop in any baby under stress as, for example, in the respiratory distress syndrome, congestive cardiac failure or following exchange blood transfusion. It may be found in babies of diabetic mothers and also in other infants heavier than the 90th centile.

2 Hypocalcaemia is considered to be the probable cause of convulsions if the serum calcium level is below 1.8 mmol/l (7 mg/100 ml). However, not all babies with low serum calcium levels have symptoms and hypocalcaemia may be present when the convulsions have a different aetiology.

An early type of hypocalcaemia occurs between 36 and 72 h of life in some severely ill pre-term infants and occasionally in full term infants who have had severe perinatal anoxia. Infants receiving full cream cow's milk preparations are liable to develop hypocalcaemia particularly in the second half of the 1st week of life, due to loss of calcium with ingested unabsorbed fat, and also due to the high phosphate content of the feed at a time when the infant's parathyroid function is likely to be immature.

3 Cerebral trauma. Anoxia is the commonest cause and may develop before, during and after delivery. Intracranial haemorrhage due to birth injury is less common and is often associated with the rapid delivery of a pre-term infant. Rarely, isolated subdural haemorrhage is a cause of convulsions.

4 Meningitis. *E.coli* and group B streptococci are the most common pathogens associated with pyogenic meningitis in the newborn. Lymphocytic meningitis may be due to infection with toxoplasma, cytomegalovirus, rubella or herpes simplex virus.

5 Low serum sodium level which may be due to excessive intravenous fluids containing no sodium chloride.

CLINICAL FEATURES

Often the convulsion has ceased by the time the baby is seen by a doctor. A brisk Moro reflex may be misinterpreted as a convulsion by an inexperienced observer, and jerky movements in a normal baby may be mistaken for twitching. The convulsion itself may not be witnessed but apnoea or cyanosis may indicate that it had occurred. In doubtful cases it is safer to investigate the baby on the assumption that there has been a convulsion. The movements are usually generalised but may involve only one limb, the face or tongue.

MANAGEMENT OF SPECIFIC CAUSES

Hypoglycaemia

If the Dextrostix test result is below 1.4 mmol/l (25 mg/100 ml) hypoglycaemia *may* be present. A blood sample from a heel prick or vein is taken into a fluoride tube for the laboratory to check the blood glucose. *Immediately* 2–4 ml of 20% glucose/kg body weight is given intravenously slowly by a scalp or limb vein.

Hypoglycaemia accompanied by fits is treated with both intravenous glucose and continuous intragastric milk. 10% glucose is given intravenously at a rate of 30 ml/kg body weight in 24 h using a constant infusion or syringe pump. A feeding tube is passed into the stomach and a full strength milk is given as a continuous drip at 60 ml/kg body weight in each 24 h. The infant is nursed prone to prevent aspiration of pharyngeal fluid. Intravenous glucose should be gradually reduced over at least 24 h with 3-hourly Dextrostix tests carried out over this period. If an intravenous infusion of glucose is stopped suddenly by accident, severe reactive hypoglycaemia may follow and cause mental retardation.

Asymptomatic hypoglycaemia has a good prognosis and the treatment is intragastric milk by continuous infusion but the volume of milk should be increased by 25% to raise the blood glucose level. Oral or intravenous glucose should only be prescribed on the advice of a senior member of the unit. It should be noted that the lower normal range of blood glucose levels in the newborn can only be measured accurately by including special autoanalyser standards. When only adult standards are used the method may not be capable of producing optimal results.

Hypocalcaemia and hypomagnesaemia

If the blood glucose level is normal, blood is taken for emergency plasma calcium estimation. If the plasma calcium level is lower than 1.8 mmol/l (7 mg/100 ml) treatment depends on whether the convulsions are still occurring or recur after the result has been received. If the convulsions have ceased 2 ml of 10% calcium gluconate are added to each feed which should be either human or low solute milk. The calcium gluconate should be added to the feed and not given directly to the infant. The total dose in 24 h should not exceed 12 ml of calcium gluconate otherwise diarrhoea may occur.

If the convulsions are continuing when the result of a low plasma calcium level is received, 10% calcium gluconate is diluted to 2.5% with 5% glucose solution and is given slowly intravenously into a scalp or limb vein until the convulsions cease or a maximum of 4 ml/kg body weight of the 2.5% diluted solution has been given. The heart rate is monitored with a stethoscope or cardiac monitor during the procedure and the injection is stopped if bradycardia occurs. Calcium gluconate is then added to the feeds until the plasma calcium level rises to normal.

The babies in some units have a high incidence of low plasma magnesium levels associated with fits but other units do not appear to have this problem. If there are recurrent fits or the plasma calcium level does not rise despite supplementary calcium gluconate the plasma magnesium level should be estimated. If the plasma magnesium level is less than 0.6 mmol/l (1.5 mg/100 ml) intramuscular magnesium sulphate is given. The dose is 0.5 ml/kg of a 10% solution given intramuscularly 6-hourly until the plasma magnesium level returns to normal. The plasma level must be repeated after two doses as the main toxic effect is hypotonia which can be reversed by intravenous calcium gluconate, if the symptoms are severe.

In a few units full term infants are still receiving full cream milk preparations. The hypocalcaemic convulsions which may occur in these infants during the second half of the 1st week of life can be effectively treated with *magnesium* alone.

Hypoglycaemia and hypocalcaemia may be found together, especially in infants of diabetic mothers, but hypoglycaemia is the more dangerous. Symptomatic hypoglycaemia may be followed by mental impairment but acute symptomatic hypocalcaemia or hypomagnesaemia has an excellent prognosis, although enamel hypoplasia, which predisposes to dental caries, is a late complication of hypocalcaemia. Intravenous glucose is not hazardous but intravenous calcium salts can lead to cardiac arrest. If a calcium solution infiltrates the tissues outside a vein extensive tissue necrosis may occur.

Cerebral lesions

If the plasma glucose and calcium levels are normal a paediatrician is informed and he decides whether a lumbar puncture should be performed. Features suggestive of a cerebral lesion are lethargy, raised anterior fontanelle tension, periodic breathing, bradycardia and fundal haemorrhages. However, meningitis can be present with no specific symptoms or signs and haemorrhages may be seen in the fundi of an infant with no other abnormalities. In the newborn the CSF is often xanthochromic and has a protein level up to 0.8 g/l (80 mg/100 ml). Pre-term infants may have higher protein levels and further advice may be necessary to interpret the results. There is no significance in finding up to ten red cells and 30×10^9/l white cells. If there is an increase in pus cells a Gram stain is performed on the centrifuged deposit and a culture set up. If there is a high lymphocyte count, serum from the mother and infant are sent for the toxoplasma dye test and antibody titres to cytomegalovirus and rubella virus. A throat swab and *very* fresh urine sample from the infant in a special medium are sent for cultures for the cytomegalovirus, rubella virus and herpes simplex virus.

For management of cerebral birth trauma see p.40.

MANAGEMENT OF CONVULSIONS

The infant is placed on his side and the airway is cleared by suction of the pharynx under direct vision. Oxygen is given in high concentration with a funnel until convulsions cease. The baby is nursed in an incubator to improve observation. If convulsions are still occurring or recur after hypoglycaemia has been excluded by the Dextrostix test, paraldehyde is given (see p.40) while the results of the detailed investigations are awaited. If the final diagnosis is cerebral birth trauma, phenytoin or phenobarbitone is given for about 48 h (see p.40). Diazepam should be reserved for convulsions resistant to these drugs as respiratory centre depression can easily follow.

If the convulsions are not controlled by a single dose of paraldehyde, advice should be sought regarding rare causes of convulsions, including organic acidaemia, pyridoxine deficiency or cerebral haemorrhage.

CHAPTER THIRTEEN

Jaundice

DEFINITION

Yellow colour of the skin due to bilirubin.

DANGER

Damage to brain cells of basal ganglia and brain stem by high levels of fat soluble unconjugated bilirubin causing kernicterus which is followed by death or cerebral palsy.

PHYSIOLOGY

Red cell breakdown

↓

Unconjugated bilirubin
(fat soluble and binds with protein)

↓ Glucuronyl transferase system of enzymes (in liver)

Conjugated bilirubin
(water soluble and does not bind with protein)

↓

Bile

CAUSES

Hepatic immaturity ('physiological')

This is common in pre-term infants although it also occurs in full term babies. Temporary deficiency of glucuronyl transferase reduces the rate of conjugation of bilirubin with consequent retention of unconjugated bilirubin. In full term infants jaundice appears *after* the first 24 h following birth and reaches a peak on the 4th or 5th day. In pre-term infants it usually begins 48 h after birth, and may last up to 2 weeks.

Red cell incompatibility

Jaundice appears within 24 h of birth, and the main causes are:

1 Incompatible Rhesus grouping.

2 Incompatible ABO grouping. The mother's blood is group O and the infant's group A, or less commonly group B.

Infection

1 Septicaemia (see p.101). Especially liable to be present if jaundice appears after the 4th day of life, but is a possibility in any infant who appears *ill.* It may follow an exchange transfusion.
2 Urinary tract infection can present with jaundice of hepatic origin.
3 Virus hepatitis due to intrauterine infection. The stools are pale, the urine is dark, and the plasma bilirubin is mainly conjugated.

Breast milk

A low fluid intake in the first few days of life is common in breast-fed infants and may be responsible for moderate jaundice which resolves at the end of the 1st week when lactation is established. A very small proportion of these infants have moderate jaundice which persists for several weeks or even up to 2 or 3 months. An abnormal progesterone has been demonstrated in the milk of some of the mothers. The diseases mentioned in the previous section should be excluded and the mother advised to continue breast feeding. If breast feeding is stopped for 24–48 h the infant's plasma bilirubin level falls abruptly and does *not* usually rise on the return to breast feeding. Although the mother can continue lactation by expressing her milk during this diagnostic test, there is a risk that breast feeding will not be resumed.

Rare causes

1 Atresia of bile ducts. As it is impossible to differentiate hepatitis from atresia of the bile ducts by clinical or biochemical means, open liver biopsy and cholangiography should be carried out at the age of 6 weeks if obstructive jaundice persists.
2 Cretinism. Physiological jaundice is prolonged. The plasma thyroxine level (T4) is reduced but the higher normal range in the newborn should be noted (see p.131). If thyroid stimulating hormone (TSH) assays are readily

available they may be a better screening test than plasma T4 levels.

3 Galactosaemia. *Clinitest* on urine is positive but the Clinistix test is usually negative. The diagnosis is confirmed by the estimation of galactose phosphate in the red cells.

4 Glucose-6-phosphate dehydrogenase deficiency. Parents of Mediterranean, African or Chinese stock. This hereditary red cell enzyme defect is found in babies with haemolytic episodes often without the usual precipitating factors of drugs or infection. The enzyme is required for the maintenance of the stability of the red cell membrane.

MANAGEMENT

Jaundice starting in the first 24 hours

This must be considered to be due to blood group incompatibility with a high risk of kernicterus until proved otherwise. The following investigations are performed. Blood groups of mother and infant; haemoglobin level, direct Coombs' test and plasma bilirubin level on the infant.

If the mother is rhesus negative, the infant rhesus positive and the Coombs' test is positive, jaundice is due to rhesus incompatibility. Urgent exchange transfusion may be indicated in severely affected infants (see p.80). The plasma bilirubin estimation is repeated at 5- to 8-hourly intervals and the results plotted on a special chart (Fig.5). If the rate of increase in the plasma bilirubin suggests that the level will approach 340 μmol/l (20 mg/100 ml) before the next estimation, suitable blood is crossmatched for exchange transfusion. Phototherapy (see p.92) and increasing the fluid intake by the addition of small amounts of plain water to the feeds may reduce the rate at which the plasma bilirubin level rises.

The blood required for exchange transfusion must be rhesus negative, compatible with the mother's blood, and less than 48 h old. The volume needed is 175 ml/kg body weight of the infant (i.e. twice the infant's blood volume), and, if citrated, it is *partially* packed by removing 100 ml of plasma from each bag of blood.

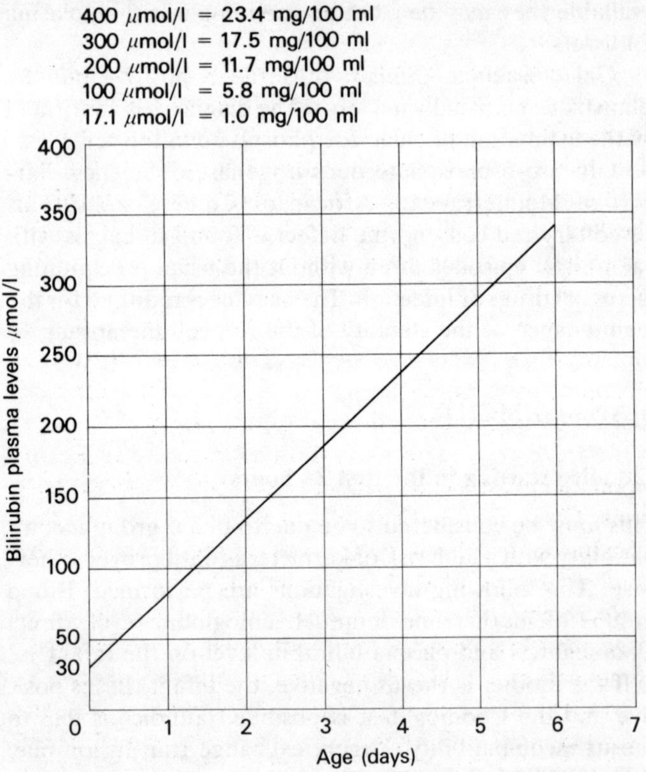

Fig. 5. Plasma bilirubin levels. Infants with plasma bilirubin levels below the line are unlikely to require any treatment (from *Arch. Dis. Childh.* **53**, 1978, by kind permission of the editor, Dr H.V.L. Finlay and Dr S.M. Tucker).

The umbilical vein can usually be used for transfusion until 1 week after birth. The catheter is secured at the umbilicus by a suture to avoid movement. Some authorities recommend that before starting the transfusion, the venous pressure should be measured by raising the umbilical catheter to the vertical position. This involves an unnecessary risk of air embolism, but we commence by withdrawing 20 ml of blood slowly from a severely affected infant. The rate of the exchange transfusion varies with the weight of the infant but the procedure should take at least 2 h in all infants. In oedematous infants it may be preferable to perform a half volume transfusion (90 ml/kg). Withdrawal of blood too fast is the most hazardous part of the procedure. It can cause a progressive fall in blood pressure which may be one factor contributing to necrotising enterocolitis. It has been suggested that injecting the blood too fast is also an important factor contributing to necrotising enterocolitis. If there is a marked increase in heart rate or respiratory rate during the transfusion, the infant's temperature should be checked. If there is no pyrexia, the transfusion is stopped for 15 min and then continued more slowly.

We no longer use a blood warming coil as there is a possibility that it also is a factor in the aetiology of necrotising intestinal lesions. We have stopped giving calcium gluconate as it causes an insignificant rise in the plasma ionised calcium level and is hazardous (see p. 85).

Before and after the transfusion a sample of venous blood is kept for haemoglobin and plasma bilirubin estimations. Cloxacillin and gentamicin are given if a previous transfusion has been performed or the procedure has involved a great deal of manipulation.

Necrotising enterocolitis with ischaemic lesions of the large, and less commonly the small intestine, may be a complication of umbilical vessel catheterisation (see p. 61). These lesions sometimes perforate. During the day after umbilical catheterisation there is abdominal distension, vomiting of bile-stained fluid and there may be passage of blood *per rectum*. Plain radiographs of the abdomen in the erect, supine and lateral positions should be taken as a matter of urgency and the infant seen by a surgeon without delay. The main indication for surgery is perforation of the intestine.

Exchange transfusion is rarely required for ABO incompatibility, which is often a presumptive diagnosis as the direct Coombs' test is usually negative. Raised titres of anti-A or anti-B haemolysins in the mother's blood help to confirm the diagnosis but these tests cannot be carried out as an emergency. In such cases, if the infant is born at term, the plasma bilirubin level usually rises slowly but the advice of a paediatrician should be sought if the plasma bilirubin level rises rapidly or approaches 340 μmol/l. If exchange transfusion is required for ABO incompatibility it is preferable to use group O cells in group AB plasma. When this is not readily available group O blood should be used.

Jaundice starting after first 24 hours

The possibility of septicaemia should be considered in any ill baby. If there is any doubt as to whether the jaundice began before or after 24 h of life, the possibility of blood group incompatibility should be investigated.

The plasma bilirubin level of any jaundiced infant can be measured easily on a ward bilirubinometer using a small specimen of blood obtained by heel prick (see p. 112). The result is plotted on the chart in Fig.5. A second estimation is performed 6 h later and entered on the table. As plasma bilirubin levels increase in a linear fashion, later maximum levels can be predicted. Infants with levels lying below the printed line on the chart are unlikely to require any treatment. Phototherapy may be indicated for infants with levels above the line. These guidelines apply to both term and pre-term infants.

During visits to the infant at home another aid to the bilirubin level can be provided by the dermal icterometer. The icterometer is a piece of transparent perspex with yellow lines of various shades which correspond to plasma bilirubin levels. It is commercially available. An icterometer is compressed gently on the nose of the infant to give an indication of the approximate plasma bilirubin level. The icterometer is not accurate in artificial light when the serum bilirubin is rising very rapidly or when phototherapy has been given. In infants with a pigmented skin the icterometer should be pressed against the gums rather than the nose.

Jaundice starts centrally and as the plasma bilirubin level rises the icterus spreads from the trunk to involve the limbs. Some observers have found this spread of dermal icterus a valuable method of predicting the approximate plasma bilirubin level. In full term infants when the jaundice starts appearing on the proximal parts of the limbs, the plasma bilirubin level is about 250 μmol/l (15 mg/100 ml).

The rate at which the serum bilirubin level rises can be

reduced by early feeding and exposure to light under one of the specially constructed phototherapy units. In a pre-term infant phototherapy is given if the plasma bilirubin level approaches 250 μmol/l (15 mg/100ml) and in a full term infant when the plasma bilirubin level is 300 μmol/l (17.5 mg/100ml).

The eyes are shielded with eye pads held in place by Tubegauze, but the mother must be informed of the procedure before it is done. Despite these measures, exchange transfusion may still be required and the advice of a paediatrician should be sought if the plasma bilirubin level approaches 340 μmol/l (20 mg/100 ml). If jaundice persists beyond the 10th day, further investigation will be needed (see p. 88).

Although phototherapy units are constructed to minimise overheating the baby, this danger is always present. If the infant is in an incubator, the heat control should be at the lowest setting. Infants over 3 kg are nursed naked lying on an electric blanket in a cot. Some infants require an additional perspex heat shield to maintain a normal temperature. The infant's temperature is recorded 3 hourly during phototherapy and for the subsequent 24 h. Extra fluid as plain water is given between milk feeds. Phototherapy converts bilirubin into a colourless compound which has no known deleterious effect on the brain.

Top-up transfusion for rhesus incompatibility

The infant with a positive Coombs' test is liable to become severely anaemic in the neonatal period. This occurs particularly when an exchange transfusion has *not* been performed. The haemoglobin level should be estimated weekly during the first 6 weeks of life. If the haemoglobin level falls below 7 g/dl, a top-up transfusion with fresh blood should be considered. Twenty millilitres of whole citrated blood for each kg of body weight, or an equivalent volume of partially packed cells, can be given over 6 h using a syringe pump.

CHAPTER FOURTEEN

Fever

DEFINITION

Arbitrarily defined as a rectal temperature over 37.5°C.

CAUSES

Environmental temperature

Some infants, particularly those of low birth weight, have difficulty in maintaining their temperature as the environmental temperature changes. Phototherapy or a rise in the incubator temperature due to sunshine or the proximity of a radiator is followed by a rise in the temperature of the infant. Maintaining the room in which the incubator is situated at a constant temperature and placing a perspex heat shield over the infant will help to prevent such variations (see p. 45).

Infection

1 Pneumonia. The only signs might be a slight rise in the respiratory rate but there may be recession and adventitious sounds. The cause may be primary or it may be secondary to aspiration of amniotic fluid containing meconium, or of milk.

2 Umbilical infection. Inflammation in the region of the umbilicus is always a dangerous sign in the newborn as spread to the portal system and septicaemia are a constant hazard.

3 Septicaemia. There are no specific features but the diagnosis should be considered if the heart rate is disproportionately high in relation to the temperature, or there is lethargy, anorexia, hypotonia, jaundice or purpura. Common portals of entry for a pathogenic organism are the umbilicus, respiratory and urinary tracts.

4 Meningitis. Often there are remarkably few signs and one has just an impression of an ill baby. More commonly the baby has the clinical features of septicaemia with certain additional symptoms and signs. Vomiting and a high-pitched cry may be the presenting symptoms and the tension of the anterior fontanelle may be raised but neck stiffness and Kernig's sign are rarely present.

5 Urinary infection. This can easily be missed if a specimen of urine is not examined in every infant with fever. Rarely, there are physical signs of an associated congenital abnormality of the urinary tract such as an enlarged kidney due to hydronephrosis, or a persistently palpable bladder and poor urinary stream caused by obstruction from a urethral valve in a boy. After preliminary washing with water, a disposable adhesive plastic urinary bag is applied to the skin round the external genitalia and is removed as soon as a small amount of urine has been passed. Especially in boys, a fresh midstream clean catch specimen can often be obtained after gentle suprapubic stimulation. The urine is examined immediately under the microscope in the laboratory. If the bag urine specimen contains more than 10×10^9/l pus cells, bacteria are seen in a fresh specimen or there is a growth of more than 100 000 organisms/cm^3 (100×100^9/l), a further bag specimen is taken if the child is not ill. If the infant is ill or the second bag urine is abnormal a further urine specimen is obtained by suprapubic bladder puncture. If bacteria are cultured from this specimen a urinary tract infection is confirmed. All specimens must be examined promptly otherwise the pus cells disintegrate giving a falsely low count and contaminating bacteria multiply to give an erroneous result on culture. Bacteraemia frequently accompanies urinary infection and blood culture should be performed if the urine shows evidence of infection.

6 Gastroenteritis (see p. 63).

Dehydration fever

This occurs on the 3rd or 4th day in infants who have been given insufficient fluid and is recognised by an excessive fall in weight and by their response to increased fluid intake. This diagnosis should only be made after taking the utmost care to exclude other causes.

Rare causes

1 Heart failure may be associated with fever at the onset due to increased metabolic rate. An incorrect diagnosis of bronchopneumonia is liable to be made.

2 Intracranial haemorrhage may be associated with fever.

INVESTIGATIONS

Careful evaluation of the features noted above may enable a tentative diagnosis to be made and to be confirmed by a single investigation. However in a large proportion of infants there are no specific signs and it is necessary to carry out the following investigations:

1 Urine microscopy and culture.

2 Chest X-ray.

3 Lumbar puncture. We recommend a disposable lumbar puncture needle. A disposable scalp vein needle may be used, but this has the disadvantage that there is no stilette. Examination of CSF (see p.101).

4 Blood culture from a peripheral vein. The femoral vein should *not* be used.

5 White cell count and differential count. The normal white cell count in the first 48 h is up to 30×10^9/l (30 000/mm^3). In the first 48 h of life there are usually more neutrophil polymorphs than lymphocytes but later the lymphocytes comprise about 60% of the total white cell count. Infection may be associated with a lymphocytic or polymorphonuclear leucocytosis but often the white cell count is normal. After the 2nd day a neutrophil polymorph count higher than 10×10^9/l suggests infection.

6 Swabs are taken from the following sites: umbilicus, ear and throat. If the infant has never received feeds, a gastric aspirate should be cultured.

TREATMENT

If the diagnosis is uncertain after physical examination, investigation of the urine, chest X-ray and examination of the CSF, and the infant appears well, it is preferable to withhold antibiotics until the paediatrician has been consulted. If the infant appears ill, antibiotics suitable for septicaemia are given intramuscularly, after all the specimens have been taken. See following chapter on Infection for details.

CHAPTER FIFTEEN

Infection

INTRODUCTION

Although the separation of fever from infection may appear artificial, it has been considered necessary because newborn infants with infection so often have a normal or subnormal temperature.

The commonest pathogens are group B *Streptococcus*, *Staphylococcus aureus*, *Pseudomonas*, *E.coli*. The pathogens causing infection at a particular site can sometimes be predicted, e.g. *Staphylococcus aureus* in paronychia, but swabs for bacterial culture should still be taken before giving an antibiotic. Usually it is necessary to give an antibiotic before the organism has been isolated but the treatment can be changed later in relation to the sensitivity of the pathogen to antibiotics *in vitro*. If septicaemia is suspected and there is no obvious site of entry of the pathogen, it is essential to give an antibiotic or combination of antibiotics suitable against group B *Streptococcus*, *Staphylococcus aureus* and *Pseudomonas*. The sensitivity of the pathogens to antibiotics in a particular unit is often predictable and may give a guide to effective antibiotics.

Intestinal absorption is variable and regurgitation of antibiotics common, so the intramuscular or .ntravenous route should always be used initially. The intramuscular injections should be given deeply into the upper lateral aspect of the thigh. They are given only by a nurse who has been instructed and supervised in the unit. Schemes for the rotation of sites are essential to prevent local necrosis and to avoid further injections being given into a relatively avascular area. If the injection is given near a nerve, there is a danger of chemical irritation causing paralysis which may be permanent. Intravenous antibiotics are given slowly into the side arm of the drip tubing rather than by adding them to the bottle of infusion fluid.

The incidence of infection at the umbilicus can be reduced by the routine application of hexachlorophane powder whenever the napkin is changed. Infants should not be bathed in solutions of hexachlorophane as there is a possibility of absorption from the skin and toxic effects on the brain. If the umbilicus becomes contaminated with faeces, gentle cleaning with surgical spirit is carried out. *Pseudomonas* thrives in a warm, moist environment and we have attempted to reduce infection due to this pathogen by avoiding increased humidity in incubators. (See chapter on the small infant regarding cross infection and increased susceptibility.)

STAPHYLOCOCCAL INFECTIONS

All staphylococci should be assumed to be resistant to penicillin (and ampicillin). Staphylococci which are resistant to penicillin are usually sensitive to gentamicin.

Conjunctivitis (See p.104)

Skin sepsis

SKIN PUSTULES

Clusters of yellow pustules in the axilla or groin which first appear on the 4th day or later are usually skin pustules due to staphylococci. They may resemble the lesions of neonatal urticaria but these lesions appear earlier and revolve within 48 h. (See p. 23). If there is doubt, the lesions should be treated as staphylococcal pustules. Cloxacillin is given intramuscularly and hexachlorophane powder applied locally.

PEMPHIGUS OF THE NEWBORN

Pemphigus of the newborn is a rare bullous eruption which is rapidly fatal and very infectious if adequate antibiotics are not given. Cloxacillin is given intramuscularly.

Umbilical infection

There is a localised red area and a serous exudate. It may be due to *Staphylococcus aureus* or a wide variety of other pathogens.

Paronychia

This is infection along the side of the nail of the finger or toes. It often affects several digits together. The lesion appears trivial but it may give rise to any of the more serious infections due to the staphylococcus. Surgery is rarely required but high doses of cloxacillin are advisable for at least 10 days.

Breast abscess

There is a red tender swelling which may not involve the whole breast and usually there are enlarged lymph nodes in the axilla on the same side. It should be noted that physiological enlargement may be unilateral. Surgical drainage is usually required as well as cloxacillin.

Pneumonia

The signs are the same as those of any other type of pneumonia, i.e. raised respiratory rate, recession and sometimes focal or generalised signs in the lungs. The infant appears extremely ill and this is often due to an accompanying septicaemia. The chest X-ray initially may show generalised non-specific changes and later an area of lobar consolidation with characteristic pneumatocoeles which are air-filled spaces. Complications are pneumothorax and empyema. Treatment is started with both cloxacillin and gentamicin, alternatively cloxacillin and ampicillin in high dosage until bacterial results are available.

Osteomyelitis

Often there are no specific signs, just an ill infant who will not feed. Reluctance to move a limb or crying when the limb is moved or touched are valuable localising signs but swelling at the site of the lesion is found at a late stage. Blood should be taken for culture. A radiograph of the limb should be taken immediately as soft tissue swelling or a raised and thickened periosteum are seen at an early stage of neonatal osteomyelitis. If there are no radiographic changes but there are localising signs, a bone scan may be helpful in confirming the diagnosis and distinguishing between an osteomyelitis and a septic arthritis. Common sites for osteomyelitis are the head of the femur, the maxilla and the humerus. Intravenous or intramuscular antibiotics are given for at least 3 weeks followed by at least a further 3 weeks of oral treatment. The initial antibiotics are ampicillin and cloxacillin but these may be changed when the blood culture results are available.

E.COLI INFECTIONS

The use of an antibiotic or combination of antibiotics with a wide spectrum tends to eliminate all bacteria except *E.coli* and *Pseudomonas* which flourish especially in a warm, moist environment. The pre-term infant with greater susceptibility to infection, nursed naked in an incubator with increased humidity and contaminating the air with faeces, provides the ideal setting for these infections, especially if wide spectrum antibiotics are being given. The umbilicus may become infected and this may be followed by septicaemia and later meningitis.

Septicaemia

Early symptoms are ill defined and the nursing staff may report that the infant appears vaguely unwell. In septicaemia the heart rate may be disproportionately high for the temperature and there may be lethargy, anorexia, jaundice and purpura. If septicaemia is suspected and the cerebrospinal fluid is normal (see p.000), intramuscular gentamicin is given. A second antibiotic is given initially depending on the flora currently in the unit, for example, cloxacillin for *Staphylococcus aureus*, penicillin for the group B *Streptococcus*.

The serum level of gentamicin should be 5–10 μg/ml, 1 h after the previous dose. The trough blood level, taken just before the next dose is due, should be less than 2.5 μg/ml. Gentamicin should not be given for longer than 5–7 days.

Meningitis

Early symptoms are ill defined and similar to those described in septicaemia. Late features are vomiting, a high-pitched cry, convulsions, raised anterior fontanelle tension, but rarely neck stiffness. If there is an increased number of white cells in the cerebrospinal fluid (more than 30×10^9/l) and if the smear shows gram negative rods or no bacteria, treatment for *E.coli* meningitis is given initially. Intravenous chloramphenicol or intramuscular with intraventricular gentamicin are given until the results of the sensitivity tests on the isolated organisms have been obtained. Levels of gentamicin in the cerebrospinal fluid may be inadequate with intramuscular therapy alone and arrangements for intraventricular gentamicin treatment should be made in connection with a neurosurgeon. If no bacteria are seen on the smear a second antibiotic, for example penicillin in high dosage, is given as for septicaemia.

Repeated estimations of the levels of the antibiotics in the blood and occasional levels in the cerebrospinal fluid are essential for treatment. Chloramphenicol causes the 'grey syndrome', especially in pre-term infants. Shortly after starting the drug, the infant becomes lethargic, hypothermic and grey in colour due to a fall in blood pressure and may die. These effects are due to ineffective conjugation with glucuronide leading to toxic serum levels of the active drug. This side effect can be prevented if facilities for the estimation of blood levels are easily available. Until the results of blood levels are available, the dose of chloramphenicol should not exceed 50 mg/kg in 24 h in full term infants and 25 mg/kg in 24 h in pre-term infants.

Urinary tract infection

E.coli is the most common urinary tract pathogen and intramuscular gentamicin is given after the presence of an infection has been definitely proved. Early estimations of gentamicin blood levels are particularly important. Once the sensitivities are established it may be possible to continue treatment with another antibiotic such as ampicillin. In any case gentamicin should not be given for longer than a week as eighth nerve damage may occur.

Every infant who has had a proven urinary infection should have the urine examined for the presence of infection every 3 months for 2 years. An IVP should be performed in these infants preferably after 3 months as examinations performed earlier may be inconclusive. A micturating cystogram is performed if any abnormality is detected on the IVP. Permanent renal scars may be due to inadequately treated neonatal urinary infections.

PSEUDOMONAS INFECTIONS

Pseudomonas is present in small numbers in the normal small intestine. Infections with *Pseudomonas* have similar clinical features to those with *E.coli* and the initial treatment for septicaemia or meningitis is the same.

Occasionally there is a pink macular eruption on the buttocks and trunk which develops into papules containing the bacilli. Marked vasculitis is present in all the lesions and may account for the high mortality despite the use of antibiotics effective against *Pseudomonas* (*in vitro*).

GROUP B STREPTOCOCCAL INFECTIONS

The group B *Streptococcus* can cause a rapidly progressive septicaemia and pneumonia within a few hours of birth or a more insidious septicaemia and meningitis towards the end of the 1st week. The presenting features of the early onset type are a raised respiratory rate and peripheral cyanosis. The chest radiograph may show extensive areas of consolidation in both lungs or may be normal. Ear, throat and umbilical swabs, gastric aspirate and blood are cultured. Examination of the CSF is usually indicated. High doses of intravenous penicillin should be started as soon as the specimens have been obtained. In addition, gentamicin is given until the bacteriological diagnosis has been confirmed.

CANDIDA INFECTIONS

These are encouraged by the use of broad spectrum antibiotics. *Candida* infection of the mouth produces white plaques and may make the infant reluctant to feed, and *Candida* in the perineum may cause a fiery red scaly eruption. A swab made damp with sterile sodium chloride solution should be used to obtain a specimen for laboratory confirmation of the cause of the perineal rash. Oral nystatin suspension should be given *after* feeds for at least 1 week for the oral lesions. Nystatin ointment should be applied to the perineal rash each time the napkin is changed for at least 1 week.

CONJUNCTIVITIS

Inflammation of the conjunctiva is chemical, bacterial or viral in origin or there may be secondary bacterial infection. Chemicals such as chlorhexidine used in swabbing the mother's perineum may enter the infant's conjunctiva during delivery.

Staphylococcus aureus is often isolated from eye swabs. *Staphylococcus epidermidis* is cultured more frequently and it is impossible to determine whether this is the primary cause of conjunctivitis or whether it is a secondary bacterial pathogen following chemical inflammation. The instillation of chloramphenicol eye ointment or drops 6 hourly is recommended after taking a swab for culture. If there is a mild conjunctivitis which persists longer than 1 week the possibility of infection with *Chlamydia trachomatis* should be considered. The laboratory may be able to isolate the organism using special techniques. The best treatment consists of a course of tetracycline eye ointment which should be continued for at least 6 weeks.

Gonococcal conjunctivitis may be unilateral, usually does not respond adequately to local chloramphenicol and is often present within 48 h of birth. If conjunctivitis does not respond rapidly to treatment, examination of swabs for gonococcal infection should be repeated. The paediatrician should be informed as soon as the laboratory confirms the diagnosis in view of the medical and legal implications. Any severe conjunctivitis, particularly when bilateral and associated with oedema, should raise the suspicion of a gonoccal infection and special arrangements for taking swabs must be made with the laboratory. A high vaginal swab should also be taken from the mother. If gonococcal infection is suspected, even if smears do not confirm it, penicillin eye drops are given very frequently for the first 6 h then 6 hourly, and intramuscular penicillin is given until the results of the cultures are available.

Amniotic fluid studies

Investigation	Interpretation	Possible indication	Earliest gestational age performed (weeks)
α Fetoprotein	Raised in anencephaly or open myelomeningocoele	Previous infant with anencephaly, hydrocephalus or myelomeningocoele. Raised maternal serum level of α fetoprotein	16
Chromosomes	Chromosome constitution of infant including sex	Previous infant with Down's syndrome. Mother over 40 years Sex-linked congenital abnormality in a previous child.	14
Specific enzyme	Deficiency of specific enzyme in amniotic cells, e.g. Tay–Sachs disease	Previous infant affected	12–14
Bilirubin	See Hytten and Lind (1973)	Rhesus incompatibility (a) if previous stillbirth or severely affected infant (b) previous infant mildly affected	 22 28
Lecithin–sphingomyelin ratio	> 2.0 lungs mature < 1.5 high risk of respiratory distress syndrome	Induction of labour being considered	32 depending on clinical indications

Apgar score table

Score	P	R	A	G	A
	Pulse (heart rate)	Respiration (respiratory effort)	Activity (muscle tone)	Grimace (response to stimulation)	Appearance (colour)
0	Absent	Absent	Limp	No response	Blue, pale
1	Below 100	Slow irregular	Some flexion of extremities	Grimace	Body pink, extremities blue
2	Over 100	Good strong cry	Active motion	Cry	Completely pink

Most babies have blue extremities for 12–24 h after birth and therefore a score of 9 is usually the highest obtainable.

For those who have difficulty in remebering this table, the initials can be rearranged to form Dr Apgar's name.

Weight centiles for gestational age

A weight below the 10th centile is regarded as light-for-dates and above the 90th as large-for-dates.

Completed week from LMP	Centiles of birth weight (kg)		
	10th	50th	90th
32	1.40	1.99	2.65
33	1.68	2.28	2.93
34	1.94	2.53	3.18
35	2.17	2.76	3.40
36	2.37	2.96	3.60
37	2.54	3.13	3.77
38	2.68	3.27	3.90
39	2.79	3.38	4.01
40	2.87	3.46	4.10
41	2.93	3.51	4.15
42	2.95	3.54	4.18

For first born infants 150 g should be added to the weight before using the table. The difference in weight between girls and boys is not of practical significance.

(From Thomson A. M., Billewicz W. Z. & Hytten F. E. (1968) *J. Obstet. Gynaec. Brit. Cwlth.* by permission of the authors and publishers.)

Head circumference centiles for gestational age

Completed week from LMP	Centiles of head circumference (cm)		
	10th	50th	90th
32	28.4	30.0	31.2
33	29.2	30.8	32.2
34	30.0	31.6	33.0
35	30.8	32.4	33.6
36	31.4	33.0	34.2
37	32.0	33.4	35.0
38	32.6	34.0	35.6
39	33.2	34.6	36.2
40	33.6	35.0	36.8
41	34.2	35.6	37.2
42	34.6	36.2	37.8

(From Babson S. G. (1970) *J. Pediat.* by permission of the author and publishers.)

Neonatal reflexes

TRACTION (Trunk elevation)

When the trunk is raised from the supine position by pulling the wrists upwards, the neck flexors contract and prevent the head from falling backwards.

GLABELLAR TAP

A gentle tap with the finger on the glabella (the junction between the nose and forehead) causes bilateral blinking of the eyelids.

NECK RIGHTING

If the head is turned passively to one side, the whole trunk follows.

MORO

The infant is placed on his back with his head resting on one of the examiner's palms about 1–3 cm above the other palm which rests on the mattress. The upper hand is released rapidly allowing the head to fall on to the lower hand. This test should be performed gently. Abduction and extension of the arms is followed by adduction of the arms like an embrace. The reflex can also be obtained by a sharp tap on the cot or by pulling the foot of the sheet abruptly. However the head may not be in the midline and this may lead to difficulty in the interpretation of the response.

GRASP

A finger placed in the palm from the ulnar side causes flexion of the fingers and gripping of the object. If the examiner's finger is raised slowly there is progressive increase in tone of the muscles of the arm allowing the infant to be lifted momentarily.

ROOTING

When the infant's cheek touches the mother's breast this reflex enables him to find the nipple. When the corner of the infant's mouth is touched, the head and tongue turn towards the stimulus and the lip lowers on the same side.

CROSSED EXTENSION

The sole of one foot is stroked while holding the leg extended at the knee. The opposite leg flexes, adducts and then extends as if to push away an irritating object.

AUTOMATIC WALKING

The infant is held upright and pressure on the sole of one foot on the table is followed by flexion of the opposite leg. The alternating flexion and extension of the legs resembles walking.

Dextrostix test

The area of the foot selected for puncture (see below) is wiped with 70% alcohol solution (Steriswab) and allowed to dry completely. The stilette is inserted and a complete drop of blood is allowed to form before it drops on to the correct side of the Dextrostix strip. The drop does *not* have to cover the whole of the reagent area and must not be smeared on. After exactly 60 s the blood is washed off *gently* with drops of cold water, preferably from a wash bottle, and the colour is compared with the key on the test strips' bottle.

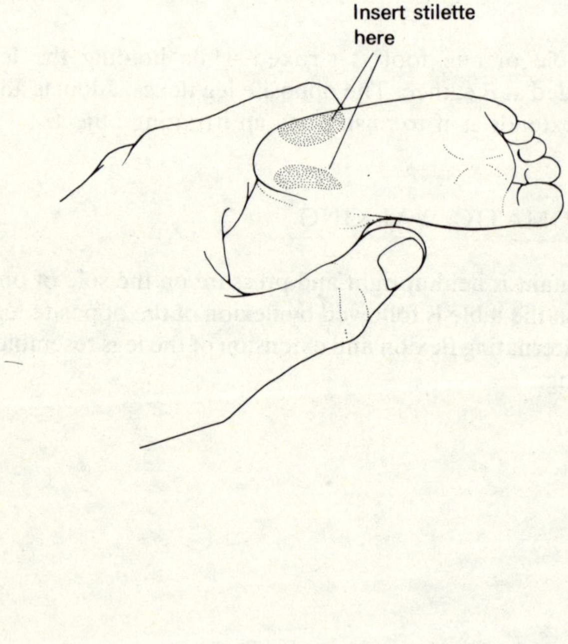

Intravenous fluid schedule

Fluid is given at a fast rate (initial infusion) until dilute urine has been passed and then at a slower rate (1st day regime). The volumes after the initial infusion which are noted below apply to an infant 7 or more days old. For younger infants one-seventh of the volume is given for each day of life, i.e. on the 3rd day three-sevenths.

Time	First 2–4 h (initial infusion)	First day	Second and subsequent days
Volume/kg	40–80 ml	200 ml	160 ml
Fluid	0.45% sodium chloride with 2.5% glucose	0.18% sodium chloride with 4.0% glucose 1.5 g of potassium chloride (in solution) is added to each litre	Same as 1st day

If the plasma bicarbonate level is below 12 mmol/l (12 m equiv/l), 8.4% sodium bicarbonate solution is added to the 1st hour's fluid according to the formula

$$15 - \text{plasma bicarbonate} \times \frac{\text{weight (kg)}}{3} \text{ ml}$$

Intravenous feeding

ROUTES

(a) Butterfly needle in peripheral vein or (b) silastic catheter inserted into peripheral vein and advanced into right atrium where it is checked radiographically.

DIAGRAM OF INFUSION SYSTEM

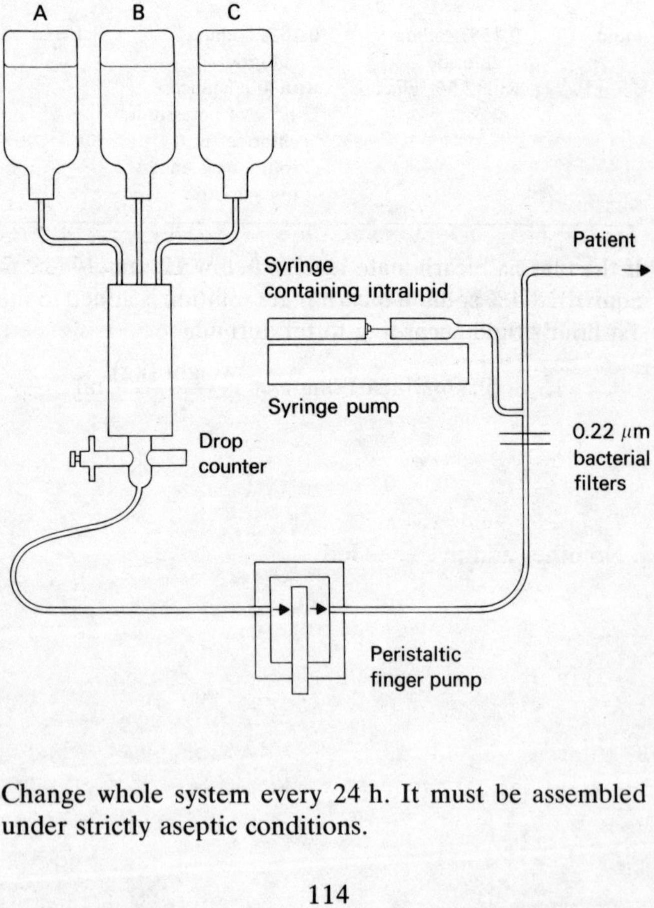

Change whole system every 24 h. It must be assembled under strictly aseptic conditions.

SOLUTIONS AND ADDITIVES

Bottle	Solution	Additives	
A	Vamin glucose 100 ml	Ped-el	10.0 ml
		10% Calcium gluconate	5.0 ml (1.17 mmol)
B	Glucose 10% 1 litre	M/2 K_2HPO_4	13.5 ml
		23.4% NaCl	4 ml (16 mmol)
		Solivito	1 vial
C	Free water	—	—
	Intralipid 20% 30 ml	Vitilipid infant	2 ml

PREPARATION OF SOLUTIONS

Mix *vamin glucose* with *glucose solution* in burette: 1 part vamin to 3 parts glucose solution. Give at 150 ml/kg/day maximum — use usual fluid intakes in first 4 days of life. In very low birth weight start with 5% glucose solution, then increase to 7.5%, then 10% glucose solution during next 3 days or as baby will tolerate.

Free Water for babies under overhead heaters: at least 30 ml/day. (Birth weight < 2 kg.)

Intralipid: 5 ml/kg on 1st day of intravenous feeding, increasing to 15 ml/kg/24 h maximum on 3rd day. Increase more slowly if lipaemia occurs.

Vitamins: as Vitilipid infant and Solivito.

Trace elements: as Ped-el.

No other additives needed.

DAILY INTAKE PER KG BODY WEIGHT USING SUGGESTIONS ABOVE

K calories 99; amino acid 2.64g; sodium 3.7 mmol (more may be needed in smallest babies); potassium 2.25 mmol; calcium 1.13 mmol; phosphate 1.02 mmol.

ROUTINE INVESTIGATIONS

Daily

Weight; plasma urea and electrolytes.

12 hourly

Dextrostix — more frequently if glycosuria is present. Lipaemia.

6 hourly

Urinalysis: Clinitest at least 6 hourly, specific gravity.

Twice weekly

Plasma calcium, phosphorus, magnesium.

Weekly

Length and head circumference; full blood count; liver function tests; plasma amino acid chromatogram; plasma pH; (plasma ammonia).

IMPORTANT PROBLEMS AND COMPLICATIONS

Glycosuria: reduce concentration of dextrose and correct dehydration. Lipaemia: stop intralipid for 6 h. Electrolyte imbalance: add different amounts of NaCl (23.4%) to glucose solution. Culture catheter tip when drip site changed. Sepsis may be bacterial or fungal. In the long term a large variety of metabolic problems and deficiency states have been described.

Scoring scheme for development assessment

External (superficial) criteria

EXTERNAL SIGN	SCORE 0	1	2	3	4
OEDEMA	Obvious oedema hands and feet, pitting over tibia	No obvious oedema hands and feet; pitting over tibia	No oedema		
SKIN TEXTURE	Very thin, gelatinous	Thin and smooth	Smooth; medium thickness. Rash or superficial peeling	Slight thickening. Superficial cracking and peeling esp. hands and feet	Thick and parchment-like, superficial or deep cracking
SKIN COLOUR (Infant not crying)	Dark red	Uniformly pink	Pale pink; variable over body	Pale. Only pink over ears, lips, palms or soles	
SKIN OPACITY (trunk)	Numerous veins and venules clearly seen, especially over abdomen	Veins and tributaries seen	A few large vessels clearly seen over abdomen	A few large vessels seen indistinctly over abdomen	No blood vessels seen
LANUGO (over back)	No lanugo	Abundant; long and thick over whole back	Hair thinning especially over lower back	Small amount of lanugo and bald areas	At least half of back devoid of lanugo
PLANTAR CREASES	No skin creases	Faint red marks over anterior half of sole	Definite red marks over more than anterior half; indentations over less than anterior third	Indentations over more than anterior third	Definite deep indentations over more than anterior third
NIPPLE FORMATION	Nipple barely visible; no areola	Nipple well defined; areola smooth and flat; diameter <0.75 cm	Areola stippled, edge not raised; diameter <0.75 cm	Areola stippled, edge raised; diameter >0.75 cm	
BREAST SIZE	No breast tissue palpable	Breast tissue on one or both sides <0.5 cm diameter	Breast tissue both sides; one or both 0.5–1.0 cm	Breast tissue both sides; one or both >1 cm	
EAR FORM	Pinna flat and shapeless, little or no incurving of edge	Incurving of part of edge of pinna	Partial incurving whole of upper pinna	Well-defined incurving whole of upper pinna	
EAR FIRMNESS	Pinna soft, easily folded, no recoil	Pinna soft, easily folded, slow recoil	Cartilage to edge of pinna, but soft in places, ready recoil	Pinna firm, cartilage to edge, instant recoil	
GENITALIA MALE	Neither testis in scrotum	At least one testis high in scrotum	At least one testis right down		
FEMALES (With hips half abducted)	Labia majora widely separated, labia minora protruding	Labia majora almost cover labia minora	Labia majora completely cover labia minora		

Neurological criteria

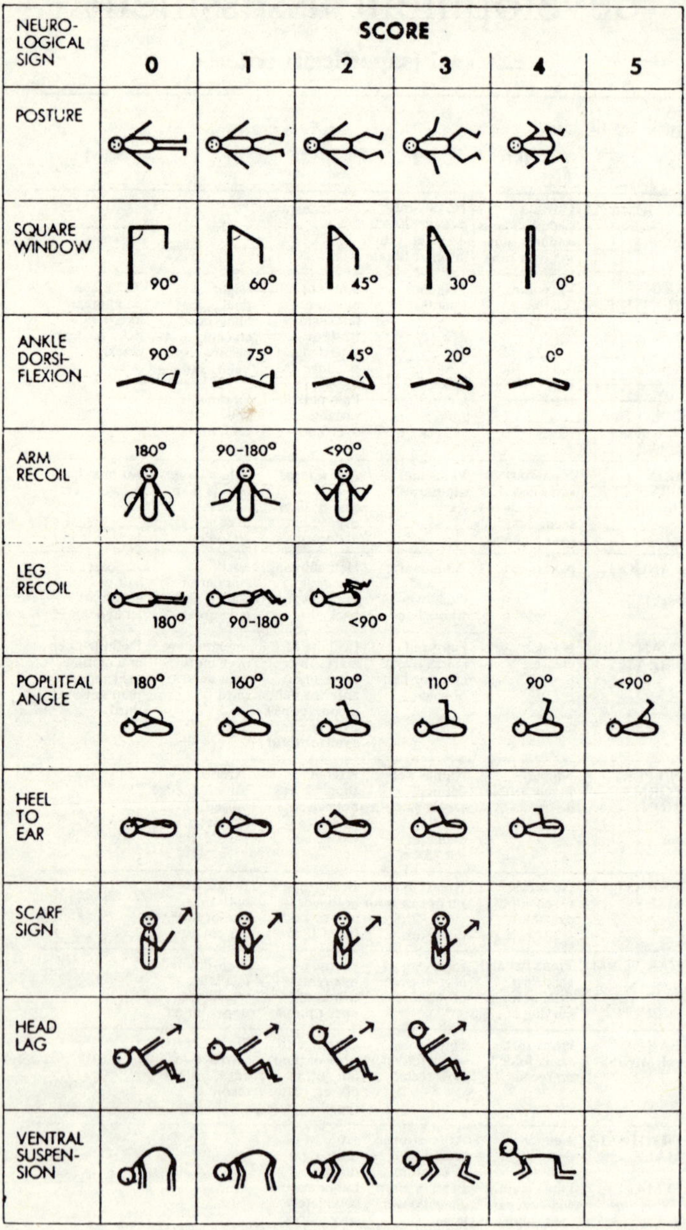

Graph for reading gestational age from total score

The total score for the neurological criteria (see opposite) and the external criteria (see p. 117) are added together and the gestational age is read on the graph below.

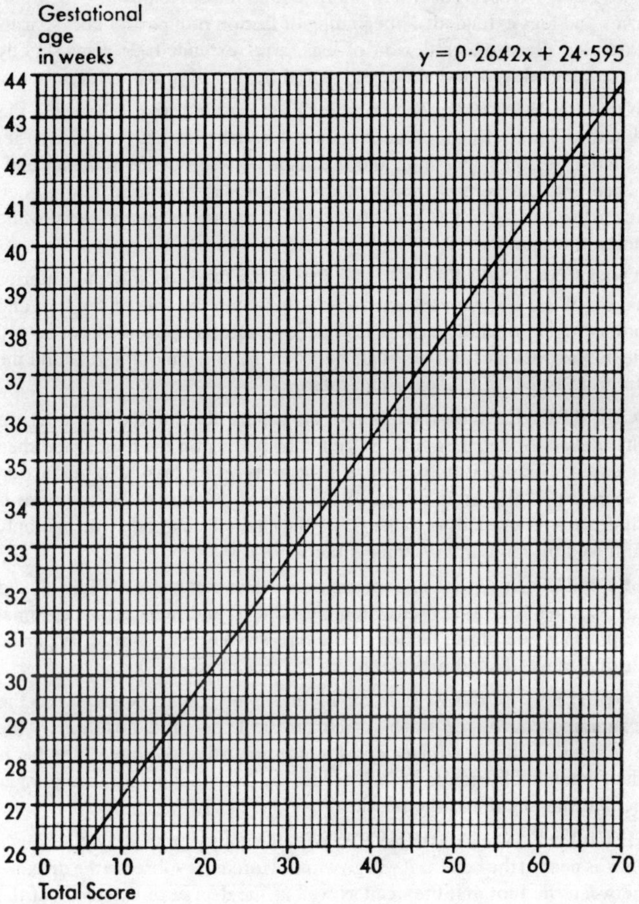

(This scoring scheme is reproduced from DUBOWITZ *et al.* (1970) *J. Pediat.* **77**, 1, by permission of the authors and publishers).

Some notes on techniques of assessment of neurological criteria

POSTURE: Observed with infant quiet and in supine position. Score 0: arms and legs extended; 1: beginning of flexion of hips and knees, arms extended; 2: stronger flexion of legs, arms extended; 3: arms slightly flexed, legs flexed and abducted; 4: full flexion of arms and legs.

SQUARE WINDOW: The hand is flexed on the forearm between the thumb and index finger of the examiner. Enough pressure is applied to get as full a flexion as possible, and the angle between the hypothenar eminence and the ventral aspect of the forearm is measured and graded according to diagram. (Care is taken not to rotate the infant's wrist while doing this manoeuvre.)

ANKLE DORSIFLEXION: The foot is dorsiflexed onto the anterior aspect of the leg, with the examiner's thumb on the sole of the foot and other fingers behind the leg. Enough pressure is applied to get as full flexion as possible, and the angle between the dorsum of the foot and the anterior aspect of the leg is measured.

ARM RECOIL: With the infant in the supine position the forearms are first flexed for 5 s, then fully extended by pulling on the hands, and then released. The sign is fully positive if the arms return briskly to full flexion (Score 2). If the arms return to incomplete flexion or the response is sluggish it is graded as Score 1. If they remain extended or are only followed by random movements the score is 0.

LEG RECOIL: With the infant supine, the hips and knees are fully flexed for 5 s, then extended by traction on the feet, and released. A maximal response is one of full flexion of the hips and knees (Score 2). A partial flexion scores 1, and minimal or no movement scores 0.

POPLITEAL ANGLE: With the infant supine and his pelvis flat on the examining couch, the thigh is held in the knee-chest position by the examiner's left index finger and thumb supporting the knee. The leg is then extended by gentle pressure from the examiner's right index finger behind the ankle and the popliteal angle is measured.

HEEL TO EAR MANOEUVRE: With the baby supine, draw the baby's foot as near to the head as it will go without forcing it. Observe the distance between the foot and the head as well as the degree of extension at the knee. Grade according to diagram. Note that the knee is left free and may draw down alongside the abdomen.

SCARF SIGN: With the baby supine, take the infant's hand and try to put it around the neck and as far posteriorly as possible around the opposite shoulder. Assist this manoeuvre by lifting the elbow across the body. See how far the elbow will go across and grade accordingly to illustrations. Score 0: elbow reaches opposite axillary line; 1: elbow between midline and opposite axillary line; 2: elbow reaches midline; 3: elbow will not reach midline.

HEAD LAG: With the baby lying supine, grasp the hands (or the arms if a very small infant) and pull him slowly towards the sitting position. Observe the position of the head in relation to the trunk and grade accordingly. In a small infant the head may initially be supported by one hand. Score 0: complete lag; 1: partial head control; 2: able to maintain head in line with body; 3: brings head anterior to body.

VENTRAL SUSPENSION: The infant is suspended in the prone position, with examiner's hand under the infant's chest (one hand in a small infant, two in a large infant). Observe the degree of extension of the back and the amount of flexion of the arms and legs. Also note the relation of the head to the trunk. Grade according to diagrams.

If score differs on the two sides, take the mean.

Table for development assessment

Physical findings	Est GA	Weeks gestation																				
		24	25	26	27	28	29	30	31	32	33	34	35	36	37	38	39	40	41	42	43	44
Examination first hours																						
Vernix		Appears	Covers body														Decrease in amount		No vernix			
Breast tissue		None											1–2 mm		4 mm		7 mm or more					
Nipples		Barely visible								Well defined flat areola					Well defined raised areola							
Sole creases		None								1, anterior transverse		2, anterior transverse			Anterior 2/3 sole		Creases involving heel					
Ear cartilage		Pinna soft, stays folded										Returns slowly from folding			Thin cartilage, springs back		Firm, remains erect from head					
Ear form		Flat, shapeless										Beginning incurving of periphery			Partial incurving upper pinna			Well defined incurving all of upper pinna				
Genitalia																						
Testes and scrotum		Undescended						Testes high in canal, few rugae						Testes lower more rugae			Testes descended, pendulous scrotum, rugae complete					
Labia and clitoris		Labia majora widely separated, prominent clitoris												Labia majora nearly cover labia minora			Labia minora and clitoris covered					
Hair (appears on head @ 20 wks)		Eyebrows and lashes						Fine, woolly hair								Hair silky, single strands						
Lanugo (appears @ 20 wks)		Lanugo over entire body				Vanishes from face				Slight lanugo over shoulders						No lanugo						
Skin texture		Thin												Smooth, medium thickness					Desquamation			
Skin colour and opacity		Translucent, plethoric, numerous venules (abdomen)													Pink, few large vessels overall			Pale pink, no vessels seen				
Skull firmness		Soft to 1 in from anterior fontanelle											Springy at edges of fontanelle Centre firm			Bones hard Sutures easily displaced			Bones hard, cannot be displaced			
Posture																						
Resting		Lateral decubitus				Hypotonia		Slight increase in tone, lower extremity				Frog-like		Total flexion								
Recoil		Absent						Slight, lower extremities				None upper extremities Good lower extremities		Slow upper extremities			Good upper extremities					

<table>
<tr><td>Later examination</td><td></td><td colspan="21"></td></tr>
<tr><td>Tone
Heel to ear</td><td></td><td colspan="6">No resistance</td><td colspan="4">Slight resistance</td><td colspan="2">Difficult</td><td colspan="2">Almost impossible</td><td colspan="7">Impossible</td></tr>
<tr><td>Scarf manoeuvre</td><td></td><td colspan="10">No resistance</td><td colspan="2">Minimal resistance</td><td colspan="2">Fair resistance</td><td colspan="7">Difficult</td></tr>
<tr><td>Neck extensors</td><td></td><td colspan="6">Absent</td><td colspan="4">Slight</td><td colspan="2">Fair</td><td colspan="9">Good</td></tr>
<tr><td>Neck flexors</td><td></td><td colspan="8">Absent</td><td colspan="6">Minimal</td><td colspan="7">Fair</td></tr>
<tr><td>Reflexes
Moro</td><td></td><td colspan="3">Barely apparent</td><td colspan="4">Complete, exhaustible</td><td colspan="3">Good, complete</td><td colspan="4">No adduction</td><td colspan="7">Complete with adduction</td></tr>
<tr><td>Pupils to light</td><td></td><td colspan="3"></td><td colspan="18">React</td></tr>
<tr><td>Grasp</td><td></td><td colspan="3">Feeble</td><td colspan="4">Fair</td><td colspan="6">Solid, involves arms</td><td colspan="8">May pick infant up</td></tr>
<tr><td>Rooting</td><td></td><td colspan="3">Minimal c̄ reinforcement</td><td colspan="4">Good c̄ reinforcement</td><td colspan="14">Good</td></tr>
<tr><td>Crossed extension</td><td></td><td colspan="6">Slight withdrawal</td><td colspan="4">Withdrawal</td><td colspan="4">Withdrawal and extension</td><td colspan="7">Withdrawal, extension, adduction</td></tr>
<tr><td>Automatic walk</td><td></td><td colspan="10">Absent</td><td colspan="4">Minimal</td><td colspan="2">Fair, toes</td><td colspan="5">Good, heels</td></tr>
<tr><td>Trunk elevation</td><td></td><td colspan="10">Absent</td><td colspan="3">Slight</td><td colspan="8">Good</td></tr>
<tr><td>Glabellar tap</td><td></td><td colspan="6">Absent</td><td colspan="5">Appears</td><td colspan="10">Present</td></tr>
<tr><td>Head turns to light</td><td></td><td colspan="8">Absent</td><td colspan="4">Appears</td><td colspan="9">Present</td></tr>
<tr><td>Clinical estimate GA</td><td></td><td colspan="21"></td></tr>
<tr><td>Calculated GA</td><td></td><td colspan="21"></td></tr>
<tr><td></td><td></td><td>24</td><td>25</td><td>26</td><td>27</td><td>28</td><td>29</td><td>30</td><td>31</td><td>32</td><td>33</td><td>34</td><td>35</td><td>36</td><td>37</td><td>38</td><td>39</td><td>40</td><td>41</td><td>42</td><td>43</td><td>44</td></tr>
<tr><td></td><td></td><td colspan="21">Weeks gestation</td></tr>
</table>

A guide to the estimation of gestational age on the basis of physical and neurological findings.
(Reproduced from *Paediatric Clinics of North America,* February 1970, by kind permission of Professor L.O. Lubchenco and W.B. Saunders and Co.)

Incidence of congenital abnormalities

Incidence in Great Britain of Common Congenital Abnormalities and Genetic Prognosis

	Incidence (in total births)	Risk of sibling being affected (parents apparently not affected and only one child affected)
Anencephaly varies with locality		
(a) England and Wales	1/600	1:40 for anencephaly plus 1:40 for myelomeningocoele
(b) South Wales	1/300	1:35 for anencephaly plus 1:35 for myelomeningocoele
Cleft lip ± cleft palate	1/800	1:25
Congenital heart disease	1/200	1:30 (but 1:60 for patent ductus arteriosus)
Cystic fibrosis	1/2000	1:4
Hip congenital dislocation		
(a) newborn dislocatable or dislocated	1/100	Unknown
(b) established untreated	1/800	If female, risk for next female 1:12; risk for next male 1:60. If male, higher risk
Hirschsprung's disease	1/5000	
(if pelvic colon affected only)		Risk to brothers 1:20; Risk to sisters 1:100
(if abdominal colon affected)		Risk up to 1 in 10 for either sex
Myelomeningocoele varies with locality		
(a) England and Wales	1/600	1:40 for myelomeningocoele plus 1:40 for anencephaly
(b) South Wales	1/250	1:35 for myelomeningocoele plus 1:35 for anencephaly

Table continued opposite

	Incidence (in total births)	Risk of sibling being affected (parents apparently not affected and only one child affected)
Down's syndrome (mongolism)		
varies with age of mother		
(a) 20–24 years	1/1600	
(b) 40–44 years	1/100	
		Varies with chromosome abnormality 1. Primary trisomy 21—twice random risk for age 2. Translocation D/G Maternal 1:5; paternal 1:20 3. Other translocation: depends on type
Trisomy 13	1/14 000	
Trisomy 18	1/4 500	
Talipes equinovarus	1/1 000	1:50

A risk of 1:20 or below is considered a low risk.

Before applying the above figures to an individual patient it is important to exclude (a) other affected individuals in the family (b) an anomaly, e.g. cleft lip being part of a known syndrome. These factors alter the prognosis and further advice is required.

Recommended equipment

EQUIPMENT	MANUFACTURER
Chapter 2	
Mucus extractor	Hyposervice Ltd, 9 Jefferson Way, Thame, Oxon.
Suction catheters	Portex Ltd., Hythe, Kent CT21 6JL.
Neonatal endotracheal tubes	Portex Ltd.
Radiant heat canopy	IMI, B & D Ltd, York House, Empire Way, Wembley, Middx, HA9 0PS or Vickers Ltd Medical Engineering, Priestley Road, Basingstoke, Hampshire, RG24 9NP.
Penlon bag and mask	Penlon Ltd, Abingdon, Berkshire.
Chapter 4	
Disposable paper tape measure	Luxan Medex Ltd, Atlas Mill, Mornington Road, Bolton, Lancs, BL1 4ET.
Chapter 7	
Model for intubation	Vickers Ltd Medical Engineering.
Feeding tubes	
(a) FG 3.5 (Argyle)	Sherwood Medical Industries Ltd, London Road, County Oak, Crawley, West Sussex, RH10 2TL.
(b) FG 4.5 and 6 (Warne)	Warne, South Way, Andover, Hampshire.
Metriset giving set V1428 (for milk drip feeding)	Henlys Medical Supplies Ltd.
Butterfly scalp vein needle 25 G (short), or 23	Abbott Laboratories, Queensborough, Kent ME11 5EL

EQUIPMENT	MANUFACTURER
IVAC 601 IV infusion pump	Ivac (UK) Ltd, Ivac House, Bessborough Road, Harrow, HA1 3DT.
Battery-operated syringe pump (Syringe driver MS 16)	Pye Dynamics Ltd, 459 Park Avenue, Bushey, Hertfordshire, WD2 2BW.
Chapter 11	
Apnoea-alarm mattress	Chemical Electronics Co. Durham Road, Birtley, Co. Durham.
Transcutaneous oxygen electrode (Huch type)	American Hospital Supplies, Station Road, Didcot, Oxon, OX11 7NP.
Nasal prongs (cannula) (Argyle)	Sherwood Medical Industries Ltd.
Arterial catheter Oxygen electrode	G.D. Searle, Lane End Road, High Wycombe, Buckinghamshire, HP12 4HL.
Fibreoptic light source	Hamblin Instruments Ltd, Hamblin House, 1 Langham Place, London W1N 8HS.
Doppler ultrasound flowmeter	P.K. Morgan, 10 Manor Road, Chatham, Kent.
Underwater drainage bottle	Cory Bros, 4 Dollis Park, London, N3 1HG.
Apnoea-alarm (capsule type)	Pye Dynamics Ltd.
Chest drain valve (Heimlich)	Vygon (UK) Ltd, Eskdale Road, Uxbridge, Middlesex.
Oxygen analyser	IMI. Becton–Dickinson Ltd, 74 Brindley Road, Astmoor Industrial Estate, Runcorn, Cheshire.
Trocar catheter (10 FG) Disposable monitoring electrodes	Sherwood Medical Ltd, Dracard, Wallis Avenue, Park Wood, Maidstone, Kent.

EQUIPMENT	MANUFACTURER
Chapter 12	
Exchange transfusion set (4110)	Pharmaseal Laboratories, California (obtainable from Henleys Medical Supplies, Hornsey, London, N8)
Dermal icterometer	Ingram, Santon Works, Prescott Street, Birmingham 18.
Phototherapy unit	(a) Vickers Ltd, (b) Air Shields Ltd, Shoeburyness, Essex, SS3 9QW.
Giving set (for blood) Buretrol FKCO 134	Travenol Laboratories, Thetford, Norfolk.
Chapter 13	
Disposable lumbar puncture needle monoject 220; 22 FG 1½ in.	Sherwood Medical Industries Ltd.
Appendices	
Blood lancet (Medipoint)	Henlys Medical Supplies Ltd, Alexandra Works, Clarendon Road, London, N8 0DL.
Injection swabs (Sterets)	Prebbles Medical Ltd, Bootle, Merseyside, L20 BNJ.

Suggestions for further reading

DAVIES P.A. (1976) Infants of very low birth weight. *Recent Advances in Paediatrics,* Ed. Hull D. Churchill Livingstone, Edinburgh.

DAVIES P.A., ROBINSON R.J., SCOPES J.W., TIZARD J.P.M. & WIGGLESWORTH J.S. (1972) Medical care of newborn babies. *Clinics in Developmental Medicine.* Nos.44/45. Heinemann, London.

FORFAR J.O. & ARNELL G.C. (Ed.) (1978) *Textbook of Paediatrics.* Churchill Livingstone, Edinburgh.

GUNTER M. (1973) *Infant Feeding.* Penguin Books, Middlesex.

HEY E. (1971) The care of babies in incubators. *Recent Advances in Paediatrics*, Eds. Gairdner D. & Hull D. Churchill, London.

HYTTEN F.E. & LIND T. (1973) *Diagnostic Indices in Pregnancy*. Ciba-Geigy, Basle.

KLAUS M.H. & FANAROFF A.G. (1973) *Care of the High Risk Neonate*. Saunders, Philadelphia.

LORBER J. (1972) Spina Bifida Cystica (Myelomeningocoele). Results of treatment of 270 consecutive cases with criteria for selection for the future. *Arch. Dis. Childh.* **47**, 854.

REMINGTON J.S. & KLEIN J.O. (1976) *Infectious Diseases of the Fetus and Newborn Infant*. Saunders, Philadelphia.

SALMON M.A. (1978) *Developmental Defects and Syndromes*. H.M. & M. Publications, Aylesbury.

SCHAFFER A.J. & AVERY M.E. (1977) *Diseases of the Newborn.* Saunders, Philadelphia.

SMITH D.W. (1976) *Recognizable Patterns of Human Malformation*. Saunders, Philadelphia.

STRANG L.B. (1977) *Neonatal Respiration*. Blackwell Scientific Publications, Oxford.

VALMAN H.B. (Ed.) (1979) *Paediatric Therapeutics*. Blackwell Scientific Publications, Oxford.

VORHERR H. (1974) *The Breast*. Academic Press, New York.

Nomograms

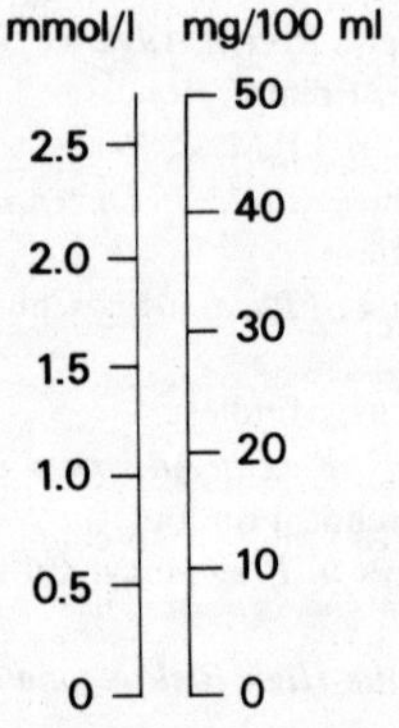

Glucose

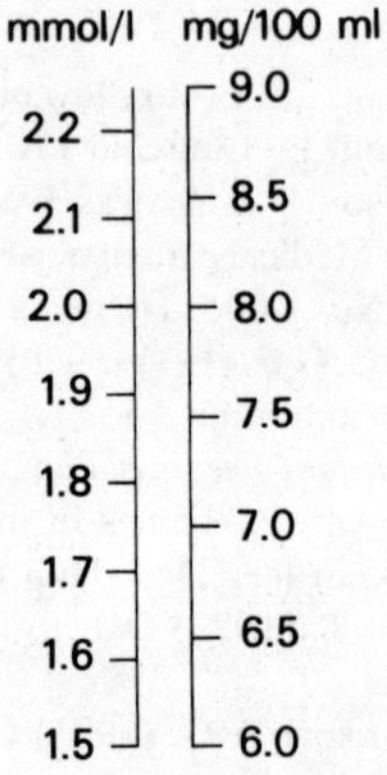

Calcium

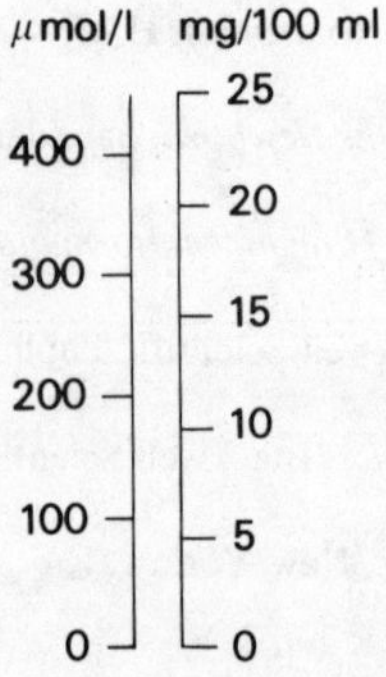

Bilirubin

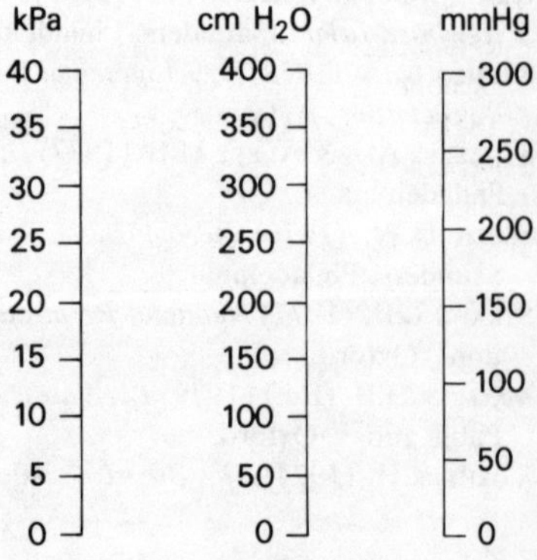

Pressure

Normal neonatal values and SI unit conversion factors

Blood constituent	Approx. normal physiological range SI units	Multiplication factors to change from SI to old units		
		SI	Old unit	Factor
Bicarbonate	18–23	mmol/l	mequiv/l	No change
Bilirubin	—	μmol/l	mg/100 ml	0.0585
Calcium	1.8–2.9	mmol/l	mg/100 ml	4.0
Glucose	1.1–5.3	mmol/l	mg/100 ml	18.0
Haemoglobin	16–20	g/dl	g/100 ml	No change
Magnesium	0.6–1.0	mmol/l	mg/100 ml	2.43
PaO_2	8–13	kPa	mmHg	7.5
$PaCO_2$	4.3–6.1	kPa	mmHg	7.5
Platelets	150–400	$\times 10^9$/l	mm^3	No change
Potassium	4–5.5	mmol/l	mequiv/l	No change
Protein	50–70	g/l	g/100 ml	0.10
Sodium	136–145	mmol/l	mequiv/l	No change
Thyroid stimulating hormone (TSH)	<1–5.8	μU/l	—	—
Thyroxine (T4)	*	nmol/l	μg/100 ml	0.0777
Urea	2.5–6.5	mmol/l	mg/100 ml	6.0
WBC	9–30+	$\times 10^9$/l	mm^3	No change

* 5–14 days > 120
14–28 days > 100
\+ first 24 h

Drug dosage

Drugs are usually given intramuscularly or orally at 8 hourly intervals and intravenously by slow bolus injection every 4 h. If only one dose is noted for both oral and intramuscular routes it is *not* implied that the blood levels are similar. Drugs marked * should be avoided if there is an alternative. We have used one dosage *not* adjusted for gestational or post-natal age as it has proved safe in our hands.

DRUG DOSAGE TABLE

DRUG	ROUTE	DOSE
Ampicillin	Oral, IM, IV	100 mg/kg/24 h
Calcium gluconate 10%	IV	1.0 ml/kg per dose (100 mg/kg per dose)
	Oral	2–4 ml added to each feed
Cephaloridine	IM	35 mg/kg/24 h
Chloral hydrate	Oral	30 mg/kg per dose
*Chloramphenicol	Oral, IM, IV	25–50 mg/kg/24 h
Cloxacillin	Oral, IM, IV	100 mg/kg/24 h
Colistin sulphomethate	IM	4–6 mg/kg/24 h (50 000–75 000 IU/kg/24 h)
*Diazepam	Oral, IM, IV	0.04–0.2 mg/kg once only
Digoxin	Oral, IM	*Digitalising dose* (safe dosage for newborn) 0.02 mg/kg once 0.01 mg/kg 8 hourly twice *Maintenance* less than 1 week old 0.01 mg/kg daily more than 1 week old 0.02 mg/kg daily reduce dose by 30% in pre-term infants
Erythromycin	Oral	25–40 mg/kg/24 h
	IV	10 mg/kg/24 h
Ferrous sulphate	Oral	Below 2.5 kg: 30 mg twice daily Above 2.5 kg: 60 mg twice daily

DRUG	ROUTE	DOSE
Frusemide	Oral	2 mg/kg once daily
	IM, IV	1 mg/kg once daily Potassium supplements may be needed
Fusidic acid	Oral	20–40 mg/kg/24 h
Gentamicin (sulphate)	Oral	50 mg/kg/24 h (*not* absorbed)
(base)	IM	6 mg/kg/24 h (blood levels must be checked)
	Intraventricular	1–2 mg per dose
Hyaluronidase	IM	200 units per dose
Kanamycin	IM	15 mg/kg/24 h
Naloxone	IM, IV	0.02 mg/kg per dose
Nystatin	Oral	100 000 units per dose (4 hourly)
*Nitrofurantoin	Oral	8 mg/kg/24 h
Neomycin	Oral	50 mg/kg/24 h
Paraldehyde	IM	0.1–0.2 ml/kg per dose
Penicillin G.	IM	24 000 units/kg/24 h 150 mg/kg/24 h
Penicillin V.	Oral	60 mg/kg/24 h
Phenobarbitone	IM	3 mg/kg per dose 12 hourly
	Oral	5 mg/kg/24 h
Phenytoin	IM	3 mg/kg per dose 12 hourly
	Oral	5 mg/kg/24 h
	IV	8 mg/kg slowly once
Triclofos	Oral	20–30 mg/kg per dose

Index